"This book is an invaluable resource _____ n with a cleft lip/palate, and the defin_____ children develop normal speech. As a pediatrician who treats children with cleft lip and palate and the parent of a child with Pierre Robin sequence, I wish I had this book when my baby was born. I would have felt much better prepared to make the best choices, not only about helping my daughter learn to speak clearly, but also about choosing a cleft team, feeding, and dealing with ear infections and hearing issues."

—Rebecca Powers, MD, IBCLC, FAAP
Village Pediatrics and Breastfeeding Medicine
Elizabethton, Tennessee

CHILDREN with CLEFT LIP and PALATE

CHILDREN with CLEFT LIP and PALATE

ೞಬಲ

A Parents' Guide to Early Speech-Language Development and Treatment

Mary A. Hardin-Jones, Ph.D., CCC-SLP
Kathy L. Chapman, Ph.D., CCC-SLP
Nancy J. Scherer, Ph.D., CCC-SLP

Woodbine House

Published in the United States of America by Woodbine
House, Inc., 6510 Bells Mill Road, Bethesda, MD 20817. 800-843-7323.
www.woodbinehouse.com

The illustrations on the following pages are by Olivia Petersen: 4, 38, 49, 61,
67, 68, 134, 137, 145, 147, 154

Library of Congress Cataloging-in-Publication Data

Hardin-Jones, Mary A.
  Children with cleft lip and palate : a parents' guide to early speech-language development and treatment / Mary A. Hardin-Jones, Kathy L. Chapman, and Nancy J. Scherer.
     pages cm
  Includes bibliographical references and index.
  ISBN 978-1-60613-210-4 (pbk.)
  1. Cleft palate children--Rehabilitation. 2. Cleft lip--Treatment. 3. Speech
therapy for children. 4. Parent and child. I. Chapman, Kathy L. II. Scherer,
Nancy J. III. Title.
  RJ496.S7H37 2015
  618.92'855--dc23
                                                                  2015024797

Manufactured in the United States of America
10 9 8 7 6 5 4 3 2 1

TABLE

OF

CONTENTS

ACKNOWLEDGMENTS

We would like to thank Dr. Jeffrey Marsh (plastic surgeon), Dr. Kristina Wilson (speech-language pathologist), and Dr. Susan Naidu (pediatric audiologist) for their helpful comments on portions of this book, as well as Dr. Mark Boustred (plastic surgeon) for responding to our surgical questions. Thanks also go out to the parents who provided pictures for the book and to Dr. Adriane Baylis (speech-language pathologist), who assisted us in obtaining them. We are particularly indebted to the many children and families that shared our journey throughout the years and whose questions led to the development of this book.

PREFACE

The authors of this book are all experienced clinicians who have spent many years studying and treating children with cleft lip and palate. In 2006, we were asked to write an article on early intervention in children with cleft palate for our professional news magazine, *The ASHA Leader*. The response to that article was very positive, with many speech-language pathologists emailing us and asking for additional information. Over time, parents discovered the article on the web and began emailing us as well. What began as a small writing project became overwhelming very quickly as more and more individuals contacted us for information.

The idea for this book slowly took form as we sought out a way to respond to all the inquiries we were receiving. It has taken far longer than we would have liked to complete this project, and it has come too late for those who originally sought our help. Still, we hope that this book will provide you and other parents with a better understanding of how a cleft palate influences early speech-language development and that you will find the suggestions we have provided useful when interacting with your child. We hope, too, that the information we have provided will help you understand the rationale associated with some of the treatment decisions that are recommended in the future for your child.

The information in this book is intended to be used by parents of toddlers with cleft lip and palate who are seeking ways to stimulate their child's early speech and language development. It can also be used to reinforce information provided by your child's speech-language pathologist (SLP). The information provided here is *not* intended to replace the information you receive from a speech-language pathologist. Nor should it be used as an alternative to having your child's speech-language skills assessed by an SLP if you suspect that your child has a speech-language delay, or enrolling your child in early intervention services if a delay has been identified. Throughout the book, we have included information on the value of speech and language therapy and other early interventions, and we hope you take full advantage of these services when needed to facilitate your child's development.

Mary Hardin-Jones
Kathy Chapman
Nancy Scherer

1

INTRODUCTION TO CLEFT LIP AND PALATE AND ASSOCIATED SYNDROMES

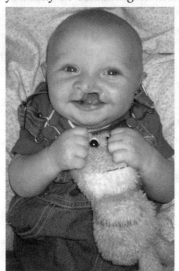

If you recently learned that your baby has (or will be born with) a cleft lip and palate, you may be searching for information about what this diagnosis will mean for him and your family. Can the cleft be repaired and if so, when? How will the cleft affect your baby's feeding? Will the cleft have any impact on other areas of development? How will others react when they see your baby?

Unless clefting runs in your family, you probably did not expect your baby to be born with a cleft, and this unexpected development can be very tough to deal with early on. Like most parents who have just been told that their child has a problem at birth, you may have struggled (and perhaps still are struggling) with feelings of shock, grief, helplessness, and anger. It may take some time for you to adjust to this unexpected diagnosis. But as you begin this journey, you should know that there are many professionals and parents of children with cleft lip and palate you can call upon for advice and support…and we will provide you with many of those resources in this book.

Because cleft lip and palate is one of the more common problems seen in newborns, it has received a lot of attention over the years. It is a treatable condition, but one that typically does require surgery. In the early months, your child may experience some cleft-related problems with feeding and ear infections that need attention. Later, problems with speech and language development may become a priority. Fortunately, all of these problems can be treated.

We believe that parents who are well informed are best able to help their child through the treatment process. This book will therefore describe the early problems your child may encounter as well as the early treatment that he will likely receive, and will focus on how you, the parent, can support your child through this process.

▪▪ Your Baby's Communication Skills

The first year of life is a time of remarkable growth and discovery for all babies. Although they begin life totally reliant on their parents, babies rapidly learn to control the movements of their body and become increasingly independent. They learn to hold their head up, manipulate objects, crawl, and walk—all important accomplishments that allow them to explore their world. Of all the achievements that parents observe their baby make during this time, though, there is none more thrilling than the appearance of the first word.

Communication does not begin with the first word. It is a skill that is refined throughout the first year of life and beyond. Before that long-awaited first word ever appears, babies have laid a great deal of groundwork:

- They have practiced the sounds of their language through babbling (and thus have a group of consonants and vowels they can use to form their first words).
- They have learned the meanings of words that are used repeatedly in their homes (and so have begun to relate spoken words to objects and people around them).

- They understand that they can use sounds and gestures to convey information and to obtain what they want (and so have begun to learn the power of communication).

A cleft of the lip and palate does not prevent a baby from learning to talk, but it can influence how quickly speech develops and will probably influence the types of sounds your baby says as well. We know that some babies with cleft palate are slower to say their first word than other babies and may be slower to add words to their vocabulary even after the palate is repaired. We also know that a large percentage of children with repaired cleft palate (up to roughly 70 percent) ultimately require speech therapy at some point during the toddler, preschool, or school-age years (Hardin-Jones and Jones, 2005).* Some may need therapy to address some of the same developmental speech-language problems that are commonly seen in children without clefts, while others may need intervention to treat cleft-related problems.

In this book, we provide practical suggestions for ways that you can enhance your child's *early* speech and language development. We believe that the experiences parents give their babies during the first several years of development serve as an important foundation for later speech and language development. The information provided here is intended to augment, not replace, the advice you receive from the speech-language pathologist and other professionals on your child's cleft palate team. We also provide a brief overview of surgical and dental management because the presence of a cleft requires treatment from multiple specialists (including, but not limited to, a plastic surgeon, oral surgeon, ear, nose, and throat (ENT) physician, and pediatric dentist/ orthodontist) and because the treatment provided by these specialists can influence speech-language development.

▪▪ Cleft Lip and Palate: A Common Problem

According to 2014 figures from the Centers for Disease Control (CDC), 1 in every 33 babies born in the United States each year is born with a birth defect. Cleft lip and palate is one of the most common birth defects seen in newborns, occurring in approximately 1 in every 600 to 700 births.

---

* *The percentage of children needing speech-language therapy differs quite a bit across studies. The difference is probably related to the age of children studied (toddler, preschool, or school-age) and whether those enrolled in early intervention are included.*

The overwhelming majority (approximately 70 percent or more) of babies who are born with a cleft are born with an isolated cleft—meaning there are no other birth defects (physical or developmental) present.

▪▪ Types of Clefts

A baby's face and mouth form in the first ten weeks following conception. During development, both sides of the face and mouth come together and fuse. A cleft (opening or gap) occurs when tissues that form portions of the lip and palate fail to come together and fuse before the baby's birth.

Clefting commonly involves some combination of:

- the lip,
- alveolar ridge (the gum ridge that houses teeth)
- hard palate (roof of the mouth in front consisting of bone covered by soft tissue), and
- soft palate (roof of the mouth in back consisting of soft tissue and muscle).

The three most common types of clefts that occur are cleft lip (CL), cleft palate (CP), and cleft lip and palate (CLP). A CL can occur on one (unilateral) or both (bilateral) sides of the lip and can be either complete or incomplete. When a complete CL occurs, the cleft extends through the lip into the floor of the nose. In an incomplete CL, a notch appears in the lip but the cleft does not extend all the way into the nose. The majority of cleft lips also involve a cleft of the gum ridge. A CP can involve all or a portion of the palate. That is, the cleft may be only in the soft palate, or it may involve both the hard and soft palate. In a complete CLP, the cleft extends through the lip, gum ridge, hard palate, and soft palate.

Although a CL does not usually have much of an impact on anything other than a child's appearance, an unrepaired CP can influence

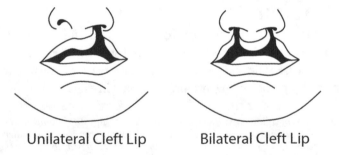

Unilateral Cleft Lip   Bilateral Cleft Lip

a newborn's feedings and result in an increase in ear infections. It can also influence early speech and language development.

A different type of cleft, known as a *submucous cleft palate*, occurs when a palatal cleft is concealed by mucosa (a thin layer of tissue). This type of cleft is not immediately obvious when looking in a child's mouth. In fact, it is often not diagnosed until a child is older and demonstrates speech that sounds excessively nasal (hypernasal).

To understand the impact that a submucous CP has on speech, one must first understand the role of the soft palate during speech production. Unlike the hard palate, which is made up of bone, the soft palate is made up of muscle and other tissues. When a key muscle of the soft palate (known as the *levator veli palatini muscle*) contracts during speech production, the soft palate is lifted up and moved backward against the back wall of the throat. This action, known as *velopharyngeal closure,* seals the nose off from the mouth during production of the majority of speech sounds (all except the nasal sounds—the beginning sound in words like *mommy* and *no* and the ending sound in *sing*).

When a child has a submucous cleft, the muscle in the soft palate has been disrupted (split) and does not function efficiently. When the child contracts this muscle, it may result in enough palatal elevation to seal off the nose if he has a shallow throat (because the soft palate does not need to move a large distance). For other children, however, the palate may elevate but not move backward as much as needed to contact the back wall of the throat. This problem, known as *velopharyngeal inadequacy* (VPI), results in air passing from the throat into the nose (instead of the mouth) and speech that sounds excessively nasal (hypernasal).

Some children with a submucous cleft have normal speech and thus do not need treatment of any kind. Children with significantly hypernasal speech, however, typically need surgery. We will talk more about the problem of velopharyngeal closure when we discuss the topics of surgery and speech later in this book.

∷ Causes of Clefting

Clefts of the lip and palate are believed to be caused by both genetic and environmental factors. That is, genetic (inherited) factors may increase a child's susceptibility to a cleft. But clefting only occurs when the effects of multiple genes interact with each other or with certain environmental factors such as drugs (medications) that can act on the developing embryo.

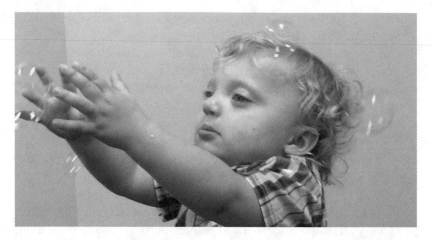

Research is ongoing to identify the genes associated with isolated CLP, and a large number of potential genes (approximately twenty) have been identified to date (Dixon, Marazita, Beaty, & Murray, 2011). A major goal of such research is to identify the risk imposed by these genes as well as gene-environment interactions. Although a number of suspicious environmental factors have been identified, few have actually been documented as increasing the risk of clefting.

Factors that have been associated with an increased risk of cleft include maternal smoking during pregnancy, maternal pre-gestational diabetes, and the use of some medications for acne and epilepsy (Bernheim, Georges, Malevez, et al., 2006; Shkoukani, Chen, & Vong, 2013; Merritt, 2005). Excessive alcohol consumption during pregnancy also appears to increase the risk of CLP, but the exact association is not yet clear. Other factors such as maternal obesity and maternal nutrition have been linked to an increased risk of other birth defects, and so their association with CLP continues to be questioned. However, one of the biggest risk factors associated with CLP is a family history of clefting.

According to the Centers for Disease Control and Prevention (CDC), there are steps a woman can take during pregnancy to lower the risk of giving birth to a baby with a birth defect. Those steps include seeking prenatal care, taking a daily multivitamin with 400 micrograms of folic acid, and avoiding smoking, drinking alcohol, and using "street" drugs. In addition, the CDC advises that women talk to their physicians before taking any over-the-counter or prescription drugs and ensuring that any preexisting medical conditions (such as obesity and diabetes) have been managed.

▪▪ Folic Acid Fortification

Folic acid is a B complex vitamin. Vitamins in this complex boost metabolism, enhance immune and nervous systems, and keep skin and muscles healthy. The Food and Drug Administration (FDA) issued a mandate in 1996 that folic acid be added to all "enriched" grain products by January 1998 to help reduce the risk of spina bifida and other congenital conditions in newborns. Many popular breakfast cereals now contain the daily amount of folic acid recommended for women by the CDC. Some researchers have questioned, however, whether the low dose of folic acid contained in these products is sufficient to guard against CLP.

▪▪ Prenatal Diagnosis of Cleft Lip and Palate

Prenatal diagnosis of CLP has become increasingly common in recent years. Although routine ultrasound will not identify all babies with CLP prior to birth, CL can be identified sometime around the twentieth week of pregnancy. Sometimes transvaginal sonography can detect a CL several weeks earlier. Cleft palate that occurs without a cleft lip is much harder to identify on ultrasound (since it is difficult to look inside the mouth with this technology).

If you have been told that you are at increased risk of giving birth to a child with a cleft, you can certainly request that a detailed ultrasound be performed to check for the problem. In contrast to the limited ultrasound that takes only a few minutes and is performed to answer a specific question (for example, checking for a fetal heart rate or amniotic fluid levels), a more extensive ultrasound can be performed at eighteen to twenty weeks to answer a larger number of questions and check for specific malformations. Be aware, however, that the actual identification of CLP using ultrasound depends on many factors including, but not limited to, the position of the fetus (is he hiding his face?), the amount of amniotic fluid surrounding the fetus, and the skill of the individual performing the test.

Prenatal diagnosis of CLP is believed by some to be a mixed blessing. On the one hand, receiving the diagnosis before your baby is born gives you the advantage of preparing for your child's birth by becoming familiar with the problem, identifying a cleft palate team, and beginning to explore treatment options. On the other hand, a prenatal diagnosis can undoubtedly increase anxiety for some parents.

Research has shown that satisfaction with the support and information provided by medical professionals does not differ between mothers who received the diagnosis prior to their child's birth versus following birth (Robbins et al., 2010). One potential benefit of prenatal diagnosis is in helping your baby with early feeding. In their study, Robbins and his colleagues found that mothers who received a prenatal diagnosis of clefting were more satisfied with the help they received in feeding their baby. The researchers speculated, though, that the parents "may have been better prepared to ask for help."

Whether or not your current child was diagnosed prenatally with a cleft, you may want to pursue a prenatal diagnosis if you decide to have another baby. If you are planning to have another child, you may also want to first obtain information about your risk for giving birth to another child with a cleft. See the box below for general information on risk of recurrence.

■■ Determining Your Risk of Having Another Baby with a Cleft

Many factors are considered when determining an individual's risk of giving birth to a child with a CLP. If a cleft condition has previously occurred in your family or if you have already given birth to a child with a cleft, a genetic counselor can help you identify the approximate risk of giving birth to another child with a cleft. A number of factors will be considered in determining your risk, including family history of clefting (number of relatives affected), the race and gender of affected relatives, and the type (severity) of cleft the affected family members had.

Generally speaking, when a parent already has one child with a cleft, the risk of giving birth to another child with a cleft is approximately 2 to 5 percent. A parent with a cleft who is the only one in his or her family with a cleft has a comparable risk of giving birth to a child with a cleft. The risk increases when there are multiple individuals in the family with a cleft.

▪▪ Clefting Associated with Other Conditions

Clefts of the lip and palate can occur as isolated conditions or as part of a syndrome that includes other anomalies. The term *syndrome* refers to a combination of problems and behaviors occurring together that characterize a single condition. Although clefts involving the lip and palate have been associated with over three hundred syndromes (Arosarena, 2007), the majority of these syndromes are very rare. It has been estimated that approximately 70 percent of all children born with CL with or without CP have isolated clefts, and 30 percent of all children born with clefts have other anomalies as well.

What are the implications for your child if he or she has an associated syndrome? In each syndrome, there are certain medical or developmental conditions in addition to clefting that can affect your child's development. These conditions vary widely from syndrome to syndrome and can range from mild to severe. Some syndromes are identified at birth or soon after, and some may not be evident until a child does not meet expected developmental milestones.

If there are suspicions that your child may have a syndrome, your child's cleft palate team can refer you to a geneticist, a professional who can identify genetic syndromes. A genetic evaluation consists of a detailed medical and family history, physical examination of your child, and laboratory tests (for both child and parents), if recommended by the geneticist. The results of the evaluation will provide you with information that you can use to plan for your child's early intervention needs and follow-up, as well as for planning whether you wish to have additional children.

It is beyond the scope of this book to describe in detail all of the syndromes that are associated with clefting. If you have questions about a specific syndrome, consult with members of your child's cleft palate team. There are also a number of patient and family advocate organizations that have websites that either provide information about or are devoted to specific conditions. For example, *Ameriface (www. ameriface.org)* and *FACES: The National Craniofacial Association (www. faces-cranio.org)* provide resources (website links, discussion groups, etc.) for numerous syndromes and other conditions.

Below are brief descriptions of two conditions that are frequently seen by cleft palate teams.

Velo-Cardio-Facial Syndrome

Velo-Cardio-Facial syndrome (VCFS) is a relatively common syndrome that has received a lot of attention during the past thirty years. Individuals with this syndrome have palatal problems, heart problems, and a characteristic facial appearance, as well as learning disabilities and many other associated problems. VCFS occurs in approximately 1 in 2000 births (Shprintzen and Golding-Kushner, 2008) and is the most frequently occurring syndrome involving clefts or VPI.

VCFS is closely related to another condition known as DiGeorge syndrome. Both of these syndromes have similarities in some of their characteristic physical and developmental features and a genetic difference in chromosome number 22. Because of the similarities of these two conditions, some professionals believe that they represent variations of the same syndrome. The term *22q11.2 deletion syndrome* is a collective term used to refer to VCFS and other syndromes that involve the deletion of some genetic material on chromosome 22.

Chromosomes are thread-like structures located in our cells that contain genes. Ordinarily, people have twenty-three pairs of chromosomes in each cell, with one chromosome in each pair inherited from the father and one from the mother. Specific conditions occur when chromosomes are damaged, duplicated, or missing. Children who are diagnosed with VCFS are typically missing a small portion (microdeletion) of chromosome 22 (22q11.2 is the specific location). When VCFS is suspected from the combination of clinical findings that are present (heart disease, VPI, facial characteristics), a special blood test (FISH: fluorescence in situ hybridization) can be performed to confirm the specific microdeletion. If FISH analysis does not identify a deletion, more sophisticated tests can be performed.

Infants with VCFS often have significant feeding problems. These difficulties may be related to a number of factors including (but not limited to) problems with low muscle tone and maintenance of the airway, weakness associated with heart disease, VPI (and the subsequent difficulty with sucking), and slow emptying of food from the stomach with chronic constipation.

Virtually all children with VCFS have speech-language, developmental, and motor problems throughout childhood. They begin talking later than other toddlers, produce fewer consonant sounds, and may not begin combining words to produce short sentences until after two years of age. Some children benefit from learning sign language until their speech skills improve enough that they can be understood. Although children with VCFS initially have trouble making themselves understood due to the small number of different consonants they produce, their speech and motor skills often develop more quickly between three and five years of age.

In school, children with VCFS may make adequate academic progress early on, but they have increasing difficulty as learning becomes increasingly abstract. They tend to have more difficulty with arithmetic than with reading or spelling (although their performance in each of these areas tends to lag behind that of their peers). Computer work and music have been identified as areas of strength. Children with VCFS usually need ongoing intervention because of the complex nature of their problems. Since the syndrome is associated with many different problems and each child may have different combinations of these problems, the syndrome affects children differently.

There are a number of strong treatment and advocacy groups across the country that provide publications and other resources for individuals with VCFS and their parents. The names and addresses of some of these foundations and treatment centers are included in the Resource section at the back of the book.

Robin Sequence

Robin sequence (also known as Pierre Robin sequence) is a condition that includes *micrognathia* (a small lower jaw), a wide cleft palate, and *glossoptosis* (tongue positioned in the back of the mouth, blocking the airway). The term "sequence" refers to the sequence of events that occurs as a result of poor growth of the lower jaw. When the jaw does not grow appropriately in utero, the tongue cannot drop from its position between the two palatal shelves, the palatal shelves cannot come together, and a cleft palate occurs. In addition, poor growth of the lower jaw results in the tongue being positioned further back in the mouth, which may obstruct the airway.

Although Robin sequence can occur as an isolated condition, some cases occur as part of a larger syndrome. In fact, VCFS is one of the syndromes most commonly associated with Robin Sequence (Shprintzen and Golding-Kushner, 2008). A clinical exam may be all that is needed to identify the condition when it occurs in isolation, but it is a good idea to obtain a genetic evaluation to rule out the possibility of an associated syndrome.

For babies with Robin sequence, maintaining an open airway is an early priority. Because the normal-sized tongue is large compared to the small lower jaw, it tends to fall backward into the airway and interfere with breathing. Depending on the severity of the problem, the baby's surgeon may recommend treatments that range from simple adjustments in positioning to surgeries that either anchor the tongue temporarily in the front of the mouth or lengthen the lower jaw to bring the tongue forward.

Feeding a baby with Robin sequence can be challenging. Even once the airway problem has been resolved, the small lower jaw and the cleft palate can make it difficult for the baby to suck and latch on to a nipple effectively. We will address some of the feeding problems experienced by these babies in Chapter 3.

As children with Robin sequence get older, speech problems associated with the cleft palate may become evident. In general, though, these children do not typically have other developmental problems, unless Robin sequence is associated with a larger syndrome.

:: Summary

Cleft lip and palate is a common congenital (present at birth) condition that is believed to be the result of both genetic and environmental factors. Although clefts involving the lip can be identified on ultrasound by twenty weeks, prenatal diagnosis of cleft palate is more difficult and less reliable. Cleft lip and palate is a complex problem that requires treatment from a number of different professionals. We will discuss these specialties and the interdisciplinary team in the next chapter.

2

Your Child's Treatment Team

Children with cleft palate (CP) and other craniofacial conditions have medical, dental, developmental, and educational needs that require care from a variety of specialists with different types of expertise. It is best if all the professionals involved in your child's care be part of a specialized team, sharing information and insights with each other about your child and the treatments she needs. Your child's team will be referred to as a cleft palate/craniofacial team, indicating that they have expertise in working with clefts as well as other conditions involving the skull (*cranio-*) and face.

Your child may need only some of the assessments and interventions that a cleft palate/craniofacial team provides, but she should have access to all of them. As she grows and develops, your child will need the expertise of different professionals. The professionals who participate on a cleft palate/craniofacial team have special training and experience in treating children with these conditions on a regular basis. The importance of the team in providing care of children with cleft palate and craniofacial conditions has been supported by the American Cleft

Palate-Craniofacial Association and is documented in the *Parameters for Evaluation and Treatment of Patients with Cleft Lip/Palate and Other Craniofacial Anomalies* (see Resources).

:: The Value of Team Care

Most professionals consider team management to be the ideal model of treatment for children with cleft lip and palate (CLP). The team can develop a long-term treatment plan that carefully coordinates the timing of different procedures that are needed, and they can monitor outcomes of that treatment. Having a child seen by multiple specialties on a single day is an efficient and convenient practice for working parents who would otherwise have to miss multiple days of work if separate appointments were scheduled.

We are strong advocates for team care but do recognize that it is not without cost. Because cleft palate/craniofacial teams involve many specialists who see many patients on any given day, it may take a long time for your child to see all members of the team she is scheduled to see. We know that long wait times can be frustrating for families, but we believe the coordinated care your child receives is worth the wait.

A recent study (Austin et al., 2010) examined treatment and follow-up provided by teams and individual providers and parents' perception of outcomes. The researchers found that children who were followed by teams received more comprehensive evaluations than children seen by individual providers. A major benefit for the team is the access to specialists across many disciplines. While your child may not need all of these professionals, having access to the ones you need can make a significant contribution to your child's care. Additionally, the study found that mothers of children receiving care by individual providers were twice as likely to rate their child's cleft care more poorly. This finding is significant and confirms the anecdotal experience of the authors of this book.

:: Your Child's Team

Your child's team will include a wide range of professionals who will contribute to your child's care throughout her childhood. Because your child's needs will change as she develops and grows, the focus of the team will change over time. For example, in your child's first year of life, the focus may be on feeding, hearing, and lip and palate surgeries. In her second year, speech and language development may be the focus of the team, and later, the orthodontic specialty will be important.

When your child is referred to a team as a newborn, the initial goal will be to provide an evaluation within her first few days of life. Your first contacts will probably include the team coordinator, the nurse, and the surgeon. The team coordinator will coordinate your child's first visit to the team and provide for any immediate consultants needed by your child. The nurse—or speech-language pathologist (SLP), depending on the team—will provide information on feeding, and the surgeon will discuss your child's physical condition and any surgeries that will be needed in the coming year. (The types of evaluations and treatments these professionals may recommend are discussed in Chapters 3, 5, and 7.)

Your child's team will see her several times in the first year of life to plan and coordinate surgeries and follow-up. Following the initial surgeries and evaluations, your child will be on a six- to twelve-month reevaluation schedule unless other issues require follow-up. If your child requires ongoing treatment, such as speech and language therapy, her clinician will report back to the team so that the team is aware of progress. Team members also provide input to your pediatrician, dentist, or other community providers who may be seeing your child and who may not have extensive experience with young children with cleft palate.

▪▪ Standards for Team Care

The American Cleft Palate-Craniofacial Association has developed standards for team care in the United States. These standards were developed with consensus from cleft palate teams across the country.

Standard 1: Team Composition. Your child's team must consist at a minimum of the following members:

- A team coordinator, who makes appointments and facilitates the operation of the team and patient care. The coordinator organizes the contributions of the team members and communicates team recommendations to you.
- A speech-language pathologist (SLP), with experience providing services to children with cleft lip and palate. The SLP may provide assessments and treatments in feeding your baby and in speech and language development.

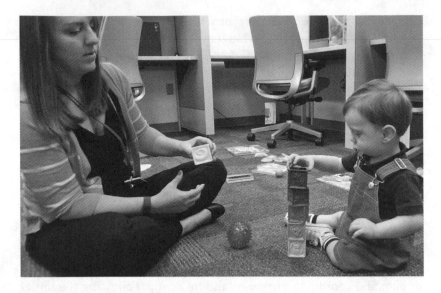

- A surgeon, typically a plastic surgeon, who will surgically repair your baby's cleft.
- An orthodontist, who specializes in correcting the position of individual teeth (often with the use of braces) and may also assist in efforts to mold palatal segments into alignment prior to surgery.

The team must also have access to specialists in the related disciplines of psychology, social work, audiology, dentistry, psychiatry, genetics, otolaryngology (ear, nose, and throat specialists), oral surgery, and pediatric primary care.

Up to this point we have been referring to teams as *cleft palate/ craniofacial,* but there is a difference between a cleft palate team and a craniofacial team. In order to be considered a craniofacial team, the team must include all of the core team members described above as well as a surgeon with training in craniomaxillofacial surgery (i.e., a surgeon who specializes in reshaping the skull or facial bones), a neurosurgeon, an ophthalmologist, a geneticist, a radiologist, and a psychologist who can perform neurodevelopmental evaluations (to evaluate intelligence, memory, attention, etc.). Children who require a craniofacial team rather than a cleft palate team typically have multiple medical conditions that are far more complex than those with isolated cleft lip and palate.

Standard 2: Team Management and Responsibilities. The team must meet regularly and collaborate, as well as communicate, with other professionals who are essential to your child's care. The team must develop a plan for sequencing evaluations and treatments for your child and discuss those recommendations with you. The team must also coordinate reports of team evaluations and recommendations and share these records with other professionals that you designate. These records may include not only reports and plans but also x-rays, dental models, and audio/video recordings.

Standard 3: Patient and Family/Caregiver Communication. In addition to providing reports and recommendations to you about your child, the team should include you in discussions about treatment planning for your child. You know your child best and can give the team valuable input regarding the treatment plan. It is important that you discuss any concerns or questions you have about your child's treatment plan with the team. The team will also help you to obtain information about local treatment resources and financial and insurance assistance.

Standard 4: Cultural Competence. The team must account for any cultural or language considerations that could affect your child's treatment plan. For example, if your child learned a language other than English first, and a speech or language disorder is suspected, her speech and language skills should be assessed in all languages that she knows. Depending on when your child started learning English and the amount of English she is exposed to, her English skills may be behind for her age. However, she would only be considered to have a speech or language disorder if she was found to be showing similar delays in all the languages that she is learning. That is, if your child is not producing certain sounds because of lack of experience and exposure to English, it is important not to automatically assume that her difficulties with sound production are due to the cleft.

Your evaluation of how your child is doing with regard to speech and language development, especially with the language that she speaks at home, will be very important in determining if your child has a "true" speech or language disorder. Depending on the particular team you see and where you live, the team may have a SLP who is also bilingual (and is proficient in the languages that your child speaks) and understands issues related to bilingual language learning. However, if this is not the case, there are other options such as using an interpreter when assessing your child's speech and language skills. The team should also provide an interpreter for you at your child's appointment if you feel more comfortable understanding and speaking another language besides English.

Standard 5: Psychological and Social Services. The team must have the capacity to address your child's psychological and social needs. This could include assessment of her behavioral, learning, or cognitive development and referral for treatment if needed. The assessment results and recommendations should be communicated to you, and with your permission, to your child's school.

Standard 6: Outcomes Assessment. The team will monitor your child's development over time. The issues important in early development are different from those that affect later development. The team will keep records of your child's team visits and will monitor her progress as she grows. It is important that your child continue to be followed by the team throughout her childhood and adolescence. Some interventions happen at different ages, and consistent follow-up is important to assess your child's needs.

■■ Identifying a Team in Your Area

You and your baby may be referred to your local cleft palate-craniofacial team by your child's pediatrician or birth hospital. However, if your child was born in a hospital in a rural area of the country, you may need some assistance in identifying a team. The Cleft Palate Foundation of the American Cleft Palate-Craniofacial Association maintains a list of teams in the United States and around the world that meet the standards described above. A listing is available at http://www.cleftline.org/parents-individuals/team-care/. In the United States, you can also call the association's Cleftline for this information at 1-800-24-CLEFT (242-5338).

If you have concerns related to the costs of your child's treatment, your team members can provide you with information about agencies and programs that can assist families of children with clefts or craniofacial conditions with funding. They can also inform you about early intervention or educational services offered in your local schools or through your state or local government (see Chapter 7). In addition, team members may be able to educate you about resources such as state Medicaid assistance and health insurance available through the Affordable Care Act.

▪▪ A Word about Professionals... and Their Opinions

We are well aware of the frustration that parents sometimes feel when they ask a seemingly simple question and are provided with different opinions from the professionals treating their child. In this day and age, it seems as though the more questions you ask, the more opinions you get!

Although the interdisciplinary care that your child receives from a cleft palate team is designed to ensure that all treatment is coordinated, it is impossible to avoid differing professional opinions when so many professionals are at the table. These differences frequently occur because the professionals are concerned with different aspects of your child's care and are advocating for them. For example, a speech-language pathologist may want the palatal cleft closed as early as possible to ensure that the baby has adequate oral structures for normal speech production. A surgeon may want to delay that surgery when the cleft is particularly wide in hopes that the cleft will narrow over time with normal facial growth and then be easier to close. These issues are often resolved when the cleft palate team discusses the pros and cons of each approach.

Differences of opinion can also occur among professionals in the same discipline. Some surgeons believe that palatal surgery is best performed before the child begins to speak to facilitate normal speech production when possible. Other surgeons dismiss speech as a reason to perform early palatal surgery and argue for later surgery to ensure better facial growth. Although clinical research is useful in guiding some of these treatment decisions, it is important for you to understand that interdisciplinary treatment often requires professionals to balance the care that a child receives to ensure the best overall outcome possible. There are different pathways that can be taken to achieve that goal, and different teams may take different approaches.

Regardless of the opinions held by the professionals involved in your child's care, it is important that you feel comfortable enough with them to ask questions. If, based on your own research, you question the appropriateness of the treatment that is being recommended, you should not hesitate to obtain a second opinion from another cleft palate team. The majority of professionals we know who serve on cleft palate teams will understand and support your desire for more information. Be aware, though, that not all insurance companies will pay for a second opinion.

Before leaving this topic, we should acknowledge that we have occasionally encountered professionals who step way outside their professional expertise and provide opinions that are baseless. Recently, for example, we have learned of health care professionals on cleft palate teams instructing parents *not* to talk to their baby until after palatal surgery has been performed. They argue that if the child does not talk, then the child cannot learn bad speech habits before the cleft is repaired. We cannot imagine anyone who has studied normal language development providing such advice to a parent. And we find it difficult to understand why anyone who has not formally studied speech and language would presume to deliver such bad advice.

When dealing with health care professionals, it is a good idea to remember that some people will freely provide their opinion on any topic you raise, but they are not always qualified to deliver a professional (informed) opinion. Be sure you consider the professional's area of expertise before asking your questions. For example, SLPs who treat children with cleft palate may have learned a lot about different palatal surgeries through their work on a cleft palate team, but your child's surgeon is best qualified to answer your questions about the type of operation your child should receive. Similarly, the SLP is the best qualified professional to answer your questions about speech-language development, since in-depth study of this topic is not part of a surgeon's training.

■■ Resources for Parents

If you are unfamiliar with the Cleft Palate Foundation, do yourself a favor and look at its website. The foundation has developed many booklets and fact sheets describing such issues as surgery, speech development, choosing a cleft palate team, and dealing with insurance companies. The foundation also operates a toll-free help line known as Cleftline (1-800-24-CLEFT) that you can call to request support and information about health care professionals in your region.

There are also a number of support groups available. For example, *Ameriface* provides information and support to patients and families of individuals with facial differences. They offer networking opportunities, host on-line support forums, and can provide assistance to families seeking information about appropriate services in their state. Like the Cleft Palate Foundation, they also operate a toll-free help line (888-486-1209).

A wealth of information about cleft lip and palate can now be downloaded from the Internet. Like most other professionals, we believe the Internet is both a blessing and a curse. Although you can find websites that provide excellent information about topics that may be of interest to you (such as feeding, surgery, and speech), it is important to remember that people can post anything to the Internet. Just because it appears on the Internet does not mean that the information is current or accurate. Be sure to talk with the health care professionals on your child's cleft palate team about the information you obtain from the Internet. They can let you know whether it is accurate and meets current standards for best clinical care.

3

FEEDING A BABY
WITH CLEFT PALATE

One of the first questions you may have asked when you discovered that your baby had a cleft palate was "How will I feed my baby?" You are not alone. Feeding is a major concern for all parents of newborns with cleft palate. Given the importance of adequate nutrition and the fact that a cleft palate (CP) can interfere with a baby's attempt to nurse, parents are often surprised to learn that relatively few babies with isolated CP actually have significant long-term problems nursing. The potential for feeding problems certainly exists, but the reality is that *most* babies can feed with minimal difficulty with some very simple changes to the feeding process.

The typical feeding process for an infant without a cleft involves a series of straightforward steps. Once the nipple is placed in an infant's mouth,

- the lips create a seal around the nipple,
- the tongue moves up and squeezes the nipple against the hard palate,
- the tongue moves backward and negative pressure (suction) is created,

- milk fills the mouth, and
- the tongue moves the milk into the throat and it is swallowed.

It is through the combined action of squeezing the nipple and sucking that a baby draws milk out of the nipple. Healthy newborn infants usually consume about two to three ounces per feeding and are fed six to eight times per day (every three to four hours). By the time they are six months of age, most infants are consuming six to eight ounces of formula during each feeding (four or five feedings in a twenty-four-hour period). Although newborns frequently lose weight during the first week of life, they regain that weight and are typically back up to their birth weight by two weeks of age.

⁘ Cleft-Related Problems

Babies who are born with an isolated cleft of the lip (CL) can typically nurse successfully at the breast or with a wide-based nipple (such as a NUK/Orthodontic nipple) because the breast tissue or base of the nipple covers the cleft as the baby feeds. Clefts involving the palate present more challenges. A cleft palate interferes with a baby's ability to suck, and so initial attempts to feed the baby can be very frustrating. Babies with CP must work harder than other babies to nurse, and their

⁘ Nasal Regurgitation

Nasal regurgitation appears to be one of the most commonly reported feeding problems in babies with isolated CP and CLP. The severity of this problem varies across babies, but some degree of regurgitation is to be expected when a palatal cleft is present. When it occurs, your baby will probably sneeze to clear his nose. Although nasal regurgitation is a nuisance, it is not considered a major concern when a baby easily clears milk from the nose, does not appear distressed, and is gaining weight appropriately. Talk to the feeding specialist on your baby's cleft palate team if you are concerned. He or she can help you identify minor adjustments in the feeding process that might help minimize the severity of nasal regurgitation.

efforts are frequently rewarded with milk escaping through the nose and excessive amounts of air being swallowed. This can result in a much lengthier feeding process and frustration for both you and your child. Fortunately, these problems can be overcome for most babies with simple changes in the feeding process. We will describe those below.

▪▪ Feeding Your Baby

Positioning

Hold your baby upright or in a semi-upright position (at a 45 to 90 degree angle) during feeding instead of cradling your child. This will allow gravity to assist the milk to flow into the throat instead of out the nose.

Bottles

There are several nursers on the market that have been developed specifically for babies with CP, including the Mead Johnson Cleft Palate Nurser, the Medela Special Needs Feeder (formerly known as the Haberman), and the Pigeon Cleft Palate Nurser. Dr. Brown's Natural Flow bottle, a bottle developed originally for babies with problems such as colic, has also been recommended for babies with CP.

The ***Mead Johnson Nurser*** has a cross-cut nipple and a squeezable bottle that can be gently compressed each time a baby moves his tongue and jaw to suck, thereby assisting the flow of milk. Although the nurser is simple in design, it may take some practice to figure out how hard to squeeze the bottle to ensure that your baby is receiving an adequate amount of milk. A good rule of thumb is to gently squeeze the bottle each time your baby sucks and pause when he stops sucking to breathe. Be-

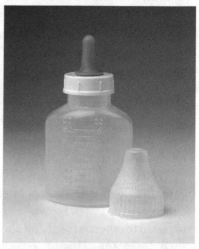

Fig. 3-1 *Mead Johnson Cleft Palate Nurser. Credit: © 2014 Brian Harrington (www.bhpimaging.com)*

cause the nipple on this nurser is somewhat long and stiff, some clinicians recommend that it be replaced with one that is shorter and softer (like a nipple that is used with premature infants).

The *Pigeon Cleft Palate Nurser* has a Y-cut nipple that is thin (soft) on one side and thick (more rigid) on the other. A unique feature of this nipple is the plastic, one-way valve that fits into the nipple (flat side on top toward the nipple). The valve is designed to allow milk to flow into the nipple but not back out into the bottle after each suck. To use this nurser, simply squeeze the nipple, turn the bottle upside down, and then release the nipple so that the nipple fills with milk. Once the nipple is filled with milk, turn the bottle right side up and place the nipple in your baby's mouth, ensuring that the soft side of the nipple is against the tongue—this will help your baby compress the nipple more easily.

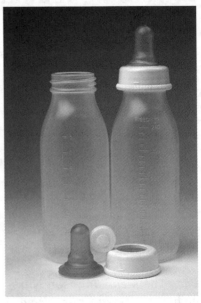

Fig. 3-2 *Pigeon Nurser.*
Credit: © 2014 Brian Harrington
(www.bhpimaging.com)

You will notice a small notch located at the base of the nipple (on the more rigid side of the nipple). This notch vents air from the nipple during feeding to minimize the amount of air that is swallowed as your baby sucks. The nipple should always be placed in the baby's mouth so that the notch is located just under the nose. The Pigeon nipple comes in two sizes (regular and small) and can be used with many different bottles.

You can control the flow of milk with the Pigeon nipple by either tightening the nipple and collar (to slow the flow) or loosening them (to increase the flow). Be aware that milk flows faster from this nipple compared to other nursers, and some cleft palate teams only recommend it for older infants. This may or may not be a problem for your baby. The nurse or speech-language pathologist (SLP) on your team can give you advice that is specific to your baby's needs.

The **Medela Special Needs Feeder** (originally marketed as the Haberman Feeder) has a unique design compared to the other bottles described in this chapter. Although the bottle is not squeezable, the large chamber at the base of the nipple can be squeezed to assist the flow of milk. To use this nurser, simply squeeze the nipple, turn the bottle upside down, and then release the nipple so that it begins to fill with milk. This process may need to be repeated several times in order to fill the barrel.

Notice that on the barrel of the nipple there are three vertical lines. Those lines correspond to different milk-flow rates (longest line—regular/high flow; middle line—medium flow; short line—slow flow). You can control the rate of milk flow with this bottle by simply turning the bottle until the desired flow line is directly under your baby's nose. The Medela Special Needs Feeder comes in two sizes (standard and mini), and the nipple/barrel will fit on other bottles as well.

A unique feature of the Pigeon Nurser and the Medela Special Needs Feeder is the one-way valve that separates the nipple and bottle. This valve keeps the nipple

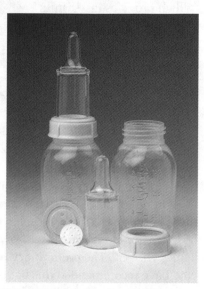

Fig. 3-3 *Medela Special Needs Feeder.*
Credit: © 2014 Brian Harrington
(www.bhpimaging.com)

filled with milk and prevents the milk from flowing back into the bottle as a baby nurses. Milk simply flows through the nipple when the baby compresses it. Each of these bottles requires compression of the nipple but does not require negative pressure for suction.

Dr. Brown's Natural Flow bottle has been on the market for a number of years and was originally developed for babies who had problems such as colic, spitting up, and gas. Recently, some clinicians have recommended it for babies with cleft palate. Unlike many other bottles on the market, this bottle is fully vented. The unique airflow system in this bottle prevents air from entering the milk/formula when a baby sucks. This reduces the vacuum effect that can make suction difficult. Different nipples, each providing a different milk-flow rate, are available for purchase.

Clinicians who recommended the use of this bottle in the past suggested starting with a level 2 nipple (which provides faster milk flow than level 1) or using the bottle with a Pigeon nipple and the Pigeon valve. Recently, the company has begun marketing the Dr. Brown's Specialty Feeding

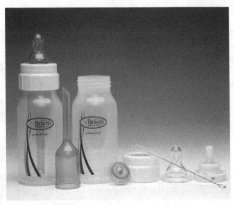

Fig. 3-4 *Dr. Brown's Natural Flow Bottle. Credit: © 2014 Brian Harrington (www.bhpimaging.com)*

system, which is designed for children with complex feeding issues, including those with CP and other craniofacial conditions. This bottle system comes with a unidirectional, Infant-Paced Feeding Valve (much like the Pigeon valve) and can be purchased in two different sizes (four- or eight-ounce bottle). To the best of our knowledge, although the other three bottles described above have been routinely used in clinics and hospitals for many years, Dr. Brown's bottle is a relative newcomer for babies with CP. The preliminary reports we have seen from clinicians who have recommended this bottle system are very positive.

❚❚ Vented vs. Unvented Bottles

An important distinction among baby bottles is whether they are vented or not. In the past, baby bottles were either unvented or only partially vented. When a baby nurses from such a bottle, a vacuum (negative pressure) is created and the baby must suck harder over time to remove the milk. Air passes through the nipple into the formula. Vented bottles direct air away from the milk or formula and allow a baby to nurse without swallowing air in the liquid. In addition, vented bottles allow a baby to nurse without sucking against the negative pressure created by a vacuum. Although vented bottles might typically be considered better options than the unvented/partially vented bottles, it is important to point out that each of the bottles described above has been used successfully by parents with their babies.

Which Bottle Is Best?

One feeding system is not necessarily better than another for all babies. Some babies may feed better with a Pigeon Nurser, while others will respond better to the Mead Johnson Nurser. Other babies may feed more easily using a combination of different feeding systems (for example, a Mead Johnson bottle with a Pigeon nipple). The feeding specialist on your cleft palate team can help you identify the best system for your child. Finally, we should point out that special bottles are not always needed to successfully feed a baby with CP, but they are helpful options to have when the positioning and nipple modifications described in this section are not sufficient for successful feeding.

Nipples

The feeding systems described above come with nipples that have already been modified to assist a baby with CP. When using other nipples, remember to do the following:

1. *Use a nipple that is soft,* such as a Similac preemie nipple. Soft nipples are easily compressed, and so milk will flow more readily even if your baby is unable to suck.

2. *Use a nipple with an enlarged hole.* Enlarging the hole in a standard nipple allows milk to flow more easily (in the absence of suction) when a baby compresses a nipple. Care must be taken not to enlarge the hole too much, or the flow of milk will be too great for the baby to handle. The hole in a standard nipple can be enlarged by creating a small cross-cut using a razor blade or some other sharp instrument. Typically, a hole that is approximately 5mm is sufficient.

3. *Position the nipple on the tongue under the side of the palate that is intact (or in cases of bilateral clefts, choose the side that is most intact).* Placing the nipple under bone will give your child a hard surface against which to squeeze the nipple and will ensure that the nipple is not pushed into the nose.

Burping

Burp your baby frequently (after every half-ounce or ounce or every five minutes). Babies with CP swallow more air than other babies as they strive to suck during the feeding process.

Feeding Time

Feeding time should not exceed thirty minutes. It is important for you to remember that because your child has difficulty sucking, he may be working harder during each feeding to obtain milk. Working harder not only means that your baby may tire more quickly during the process, but that he may be using more calories during the process of feeding than he can ingest, and this can result in weight loss and failure to thrive. The cleft palate team may instruct you to feed your baby smaller amounts more frequently throughout the day to ensure that he receives adequate nutrition while avoiding prolonged feeding times.

▪▪ Troubleshooting Common Feeding Problems	
Problem	**Solution**
Nipple collapses	Loosen the collar around the nipple until the nipple expands again.
Milk is not coming through the nipple	Make sure the cross-cut or Y-cut is open through the nipple. Check to be sure the one-way valve is not stuck (if the nipple has one).
Feeder is leaking	Check that all parts of the feeder have been assembled properly. Check to see if any parts appear worn and need to be replaced.

▪▪ Breastfeeding Your Baby

Babies with an isolated CL can often breastfeed successfully because breast tissue covers the cleft when the baby latches on to the nipple. Breastfeeding a baby with a CP, however, is far more challenging. Because they are not able to produce the suction needed to pull milk from the breast, the majority of these babies find it difficult to successfully nurse at the breast.

Many professionals on cleft palate teams will advise you to use a breast pump to express breast milk and then bottle-feed your baby. This is to ensure that your baby is getting the nutrition he needs. If desired, you can put your baby to your breast once he has consumed the milk in his bottle. If you decide to try breastfeeding with your child, make sure that his weight is being carefully monitored by a pediatrician or cleft palate team. Remember that while you can measure the amount of milk your baby is taking from a bottle, you have no way of monitoring his intake from your breast. Careful monitoring of weight gain is essential for these infants.

Your pediatrician and cleft palate team will follow your baby closely to ensure that he is putting on adequate weight. Do not be shy about asking for help if you need it. Your cleft palate team can assist you in identifying someone in your community (usually a nurse or SLP) who can provide assistance. If you do not yet have a cleft palate team and do not know whom to contact, your best option is to contact the Cleft Palate Foundation at 1-800-242-5338. They can help you identify a professional in your area.

▪▪ Introducing Solid Foods

Babies with CP are usually introduced to solid foods on the same schedule as other babies are. Once your child is four to six months old, check with your pediatrician to determine if he is ready for soft solid (strained or pureed) foods. Babies often let us know when they are ready for solid foods by looking and reaching for food at the table. Before introducing your child to solid foods, he should be sitting up and demonstrating good head and neck control.

A common food that is often introduced first is infant cereal mixed with breast milk or formula. It may be helpful to offer your baby breast milk or formula first, and then while he is still hungry, place a spoon next to his lips. Your baby may reject the spoon at first, but try again in a few minutes. If he is not interested, do not be concerned. It can take a while for some babies to accept a spoon. Remember, your baby is still receiving breast milk or formula, so he is receiving adequate nutrition.

Once your child begins taking food from a spoon, expect to see it everywhere except his tummy! As he gets adept at eating from a spoon, consult with your pediatrician to determine if it is time to introduce a pureed fruit or vegetable. Wait several days after introducing a new food before introducing another one. That way, you will be able to identify food allergies if they exist.

If your child's cleft palate has not yet been repaired, some food will probably be pushed into his nose as he eats. When this happens, it can cause some babies to cough or sneeze...which may clear the food from their nose. In most cases, this food will be removed as your baby sucks or swallows. If the food is not cleared out as your baby continues

eating, you can fre-
quently clear it by giv-
ing him some water
to drink. A reduction
in nasal regurgitation
(and thus sneezing)
can be expected over
time as your child be-
comes more adept at
manipulating food in
his mouth.

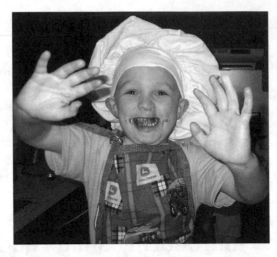

At eight to twelve
months, your baby will
probably be ready for
coarser table foods that can be cut up or mashed, and by one year of
age, most babies who are taking formula or breast milk are ready for
cow's (whole) milk. Your pediatrician and other members of the cleft
palate team may recommend that you dilute thicker foods to minimize
the amount that gets embedded in the cleft or nose. In addition, they
may recommend that you avoid introducing spicy foods until after the
palate has been repaired since these foods can irritate the nasal tissues.

■■ Introducing Cup Drinking

If you have not introduced cup drinking by the time you start your
baby on coarser table foods, now may be a good time to do so. Some
surgeons do not want a baby to use a bottle immediately after surgery
to repair the CP. Although there is some disagreement among surgeons
on this issue, some believe that the use of a bottle immediately after
surgery can damage the sutures and result in partial breakdown of the
surgery. Straws and pacifiers are also discouraged for the same reason.

You and your baby will find it much easier to continue a familiar
feeding routine than adapt to a new one, so be sure to introduce your
baby to cup drinking before palatal surgery if you know that a bottle
will not be permitted immediately after the surgery. Cups that are open
or cut out (with an area on top cut out for the nose) are good choices.
Sippy cups with spouts or straws should be avoided. If you want to use
a sippy cup, be sure to show the cup to your child's surgeon prior to surgery to verify that it will be acceptable for use following palatal repair.

Cups can be introduced when a baby is approximately eight or nine months old. Ideally, your baby should be drinking from a cup at least one month prior to palatal surgery (if a cup will be used following surgery). Remember that cup drinking, like other developmental activities, is a skill that is refined over time with lots of practice. At first, the goal will be to just familiarize your baby with the cup. Place a small amount of liquid (milk or water) in the cup and offer it to him. Although you will hold onto the cup at first, gradually allow your baby to hold the cup without your assistance. Of course, most of the liquid will end up on your baby, the highchair tray, or the floor to begin with, and that is fine. The more experience your baby has with the cup, the more proficient he will become in drinking from it.

Once your baby is familiar with the cup and will attempt to drink from it, you can gradually eliminate his bottle at breakfast while continuing to provide it at other meals. Over time (a week or two), you can eliminate another bottle feeding (e.g., lunchtime). Although babies differ in their preference, the last bottle a baby takes before bedtime is usually the hardest to eliminate and should be replaced last.

▪▪ Feeding Obturators

Some professionals recommend the use of palatal obturators prior to palatal surgery to assist with the feeding process. The obturator provides a hard, acrylic surface against which the nipple can be squeezed. Although you might think that such an appliance would make it easier for a baby to nurse, there has been limited research conducted examining their use. To our knowledge, they are not routinely used in many centers across the United States. We suspect that there are two reasons for this. First, the benefits of using a palatal obturator during feeding have not been fully supported through clinical research. Second, many babies are able to nurse without them once parents are informed about appropriate positioning and bottles/nipples.

▪▪ Feeding Your Baby after Surgery

Check with your surgeon regarding the introduction of soft foods immediately following surgery. Some surgeons will approve semi-solid foods as long as they are soft and do not contain any chunks that are likely to get stuck in the areas of the palate that are healing (see discussion on feeding following surgery in Chapter 5). Typically, most children resume a normal diet approximately two weeks following surgery. Your surgeon will advise you on your child's specific needs.

▪▪ Feeding Concerns Following Surgery

Occasionally, a small hole (called a fistula) will develop along the surgical site following palatal surgery. These holes can develop for a variety of reasons (including tension at the surgical site following repair of a wide cleft) and can occur anywhere along the site of the original cleft. Most commonly, they occur in the hard palate or at the juncture of the hard and soft palate. Food can get trapped in a fistula, but it is usually cleared when a child drinks.

If food and liquid routinely leak through your child's nose after palatal surgery, you should talk to your child's surgeon. Be aware, though, that some small fistulas do not affect feeding at all. That is because, in some cases, the hole that is visible in the mouth is not actually open all the way into the nose. A fistula is not usually repaired unless it has a significant impact on a child's speech or feeding.

▪▪ A Word about Feeding Babies with Syndromes

Babies born with a syndrome that involves a CP or velopharyngeal inadequacy (VPI) may have the same feeding problems as babies born with isolated clefts have. Because syndromes involve problems other than the cleft, it is possible that these babies may have additional feeding problems as well.

It is beyond the scope of this book to describe in detail all of the difficulties that these babies may demonstrate, but we will highlight some key problems associated with some of the more common syndromes below. Because of the medical complications associated with many of these problems, children with syndromes may need a comprehensive feeding assessment involving several specialists. Treatment for some of the physical problems that compromise feeding may include changes in the feeding schedule (for example, a reduction in feeding time when fatigue is a problem), medications, or surgery.

Problem	Associated Syndrome/ Sequence	Feeding Issue
reduced muscle tone	VCFS	airway collapse; problems with swallow
cleft palate; VPI	VCFS Robin Sequence	nasal regurgitation; weak suck
heart problems	VCFS	fatigue
slow emptying of digestive tract & chronic constipation	VCFS	stomach cramps; poor appetite
airway compromise	Robin Sequence	choking & aspiration; fatigue
esophageal obstruction	VCFS	food cannot reach stomach
micrognathia (small lower jaw)	Robin Sequence	airway compromise; nipple

▪▪ How Common Are Feeding Problems in Babies with Clefts?

Researchers in Australia studied feeding in forty-six babies with isolated CL, CP, and CLP at two weeks, three months, and fourteen months of age (Reid, Kilpatrick, and Reilly, 2006). They reported that all babies with CL had good or satisfactory feeding skills at each age studied. Of the thirty-five babies with CP and CLP they studied, twenty-eight (80 percent) had good or satisfactory feeding skills at two weeks of age, and that percentage rose to 94 percent (33/35) at three months of age and 97 percent (34/35) at fourteen months of age. The most commonly reported feeding problem in these babies was nasal regurgitation. The researchers concluded from their findings that while some babies with isolated CP and CLP may need assistance with feeding during the first month of life, these problems typically resolve by three months of age.

The researchers also studied sixteen babies with either Robin Sequence or a syndrome that included cleft palate. As explained in Chapter 1, Robin sequence is a condition where growth of the jaw is restricted during prenatal development and results in a smaller jaw at birth. The small jaw is often associated with feeding and breathing difficulties, especially during infancy. In the Australian study, all but three (81 percent) of the sixteen babies had poor feeding skills at two weeks of age, 62.5 percent continued to have poor skills at three months, and 56 percent continued to have poor skills at fourteen months. The researchers concluded that having a diagnosis of Robin sequence or a syndrome substantially increased the odds of an infant having a feeding problem.

‖ An Important Resource for You

The Cleft Palate Foundation has developed excellent instructional videos that provide basic information about feeding and show you how to use the special bottles described above. The issue of breastfeeding is also discussed. You can view the videos on the foundation's website at http://www.cleftline.org/parents/feeding_your_baby.

‖ A Final Word

In this chapter we described the feeding problems commonly seen in babies with CP and discussed some possible solutions for those problems. Any discussion of feeding in these babies would be incomplete, however, if we did not also acknowledge that successfully feeding a baby with CP involves a lot of patience. The impact of a cleft palate can be minimized by making modifications in positioning and carefully selecting the bottle and nipple you use. This, in turn, can help your baby feed more easily and gain weight.

None of this is achieved, however, without a lot of effort on your part. The trial and error involved and the continued leakage of milk through your baby's nose prior to palatal surgery can be very frustrating. Remember that while professionals can advise you on options to minimize problems you are having in feeding your baby, parents of babies with CP who have walked in your shoes are one of the best resources you have. Ask the professionals involved in your child's care if they know of a parent support group in your area. If one does not exist, they might know of other parents in the area who would be willing to meet with you. In addition, there are a number of organizations that provide telephone and online counseling and support. See *Resources* at the back of the book for information.

4

YOUR CHILD'S
EARS AND HEARING

Ear infections are one of the most common medical problems among children. According to the National Institute on Deafness and Other Communication Disorders (NIDCD), approximately 75 percent of all toddlers will experience at least one infection prior to their third birthday.

For babies born with cleft palate (CP), the incidence of ear infections is even higher, with different studies reporting ear infections in 90 to 100 percent of young children with CP. You may see a decrease in the number of ear infections your baby experiences after palatal surgery, after insertion of PE tubes (if they are recommended), or as your baby gets older. In the meantime, ear infections are a concern because they can be painful and can result in hearing loss. Hearing loss, in turn, can be associated with speech and language delays.

Ear infections may never be 100 percent preventable for any group of children. But the negative effect on speech and language development can be minimized with careful medical monitoring of your child's ears and hearing. There are also steps you can take to help your child compensate during periods that her hearing is affected.

■■ Why Are Ear Infections So Common in Young Children?

In order to understand why ear infections are more common in children, you need to first understand some basics about the anatomy and function of the ear.

The *outer ear,* which is responsible for collecting sound, is separated from the *middle ear* by the eardrum. The middle ear is an air-filled cavity that contains three small bones that form a chain attached to the eardrum on one end and the *inner ear* on the other end (see Figure 4-1). When sound hits the eardrum, it vibrates and causes the middle ear bones to move and transmit sound waves to the inner ear. These vibrations change into electrical signals in the inner ear and are sent to the brain. These signals are what the brain hears as sounds.

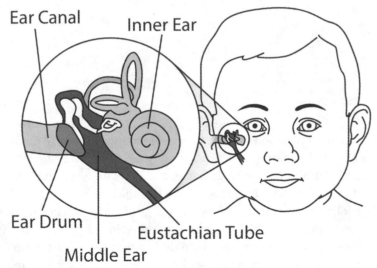

Fig. 4-1 *Structure of the Ear.*

The middle ear is typically an air-filled space that is connected to the Eustachian tube, a tube that runs from the back of the nose to the middle ear. This tube is usually closed but opens periodically to equalize the pressure within the middle ear with the pressure outside the ears. When blockage of the Eustachian tube occurs due to upper respiratory infections (colds or flu), enlarged adenoids, allergies, or environmental pollutants, fluid that develops in the middle space may not drain properly. This condition can occur at any age, but it occurs more commonly in young children because their Eustachian tube is shorter and more horizontal than an adult's. As children grow, the tube becomes increasingly slanted, and drainage is easier.

Babies with CP are at greater risk than other babies for middle ear infections, particularly before the cleft is surgically repaired. This is because muscles that open the Eustachian tube were disrupted by the cleft and are not as effective at opening the tube. When the Eustachian tube does not open, air is prevented from entering (and appropriately pressurizing) the middle ear space. Fluid then accumulates and the individual experiences an ear infection (see below).

▪▪ Types of Ear Infections

The accumulation of fluid in the middle ear may result in either *acute otitis media* (AOM) or *otitis media with effusion* (OME), each of which has different symptoms and treatments. AOM occurs when the fluid in the ear becomes infected. AOM is usually accompanied by pain, redness of the eardrum, fever, and "pus" in the ear and may or may not be accompanied by hearing loss. The cause of AOM is typically bacterial, so it is often treated with antibiotics. When ear infections do not clear up naturally or with the use of antibiotics, an ear, nose, and throat (ENT) physician may decide to surgically insert pressure equalizing (PE) tubes in the child's eardrum in order to allow the fluid to drain. See the section on "How Ear Infections Are Treated" for more detail about the different treatment options.

The second and most common type of ear infection is OME, often referred to as "glue ear" because it is characterized by the build-up of sticky fluid in the middle ear. In contrast to AOM, the fluid is not infected. Therefore, OME is *not* accompanied by pain, fever, or the other symptoms associated with AOM. However, OME can cause a hearing loss. Your child may also be uncomfortable because she may feel pressure and have that "stuffed up" feeling. It is not uncommon for OME to go undetected until identified by tympanometry (a type of hearing test discussed below) or by a doctor looking into your child's ear. OME is typically not treated with antibiotics and will usually go away with time.

It is important that your doctor determines the type of ear infection your child has so that he or she can advise you concerning the appropriate course of treatment. However, discriminating between AOM and OME is often difficult in infants and young children.

▪▪ What Are the Consequences of Repeated Ear Infections?

Speech-language pathologists (SLP) are concerned about repeated ear infections in babies because the fluid that accumulates in the middle ear typically impairs hearing. The fluid actually dampens the sound waves as they travel through the middle ear cavity and on to the inner ear. This decreases the strength or loudness of the sound that your baby hears. This type of hearing loss is called a *conductive hearing loss* because there is a "barrier" in the outer or middle ear that interferes with "conduction" of sound.

Conductive hearing loss may be treated medically or with surgery and is often reversible. This is in contrast to a *sensorineural hearing loss,* which results from some type of damage to the inner ear or the nerves associated with hearing. Sensorineural hearing loss cannot typically be reversed with medical treatment.

In the case of conductive hearing loss associated with ear infections, the degree of hearing loss ranges from mild to moderate. Also, the degree of hearing loss fluctuates over time. This is related to changes in the amount and type of fluid present. So, as the amount of fluid increases or the fluid becomes thicker (sometimes described as glue-like), the amount of hearing loss increases. As the infection resolves (over a period of a few days to a month or longer), the amount of the loss decreases until hearing finally returns to normal. In the meantime, a chronic ear infection may cause a toddler who is learning to talk to miss out on important information in speech and language.

▪▪ How Does Hearing Loss Affect Your Child's Ability to Hear Sounds and Speech?

Sounds that we hear vary in terms of pitch (*frequency*) and loudness (*intensity*). Frequency—or how low- or high-pitched a sound is—is measured in Hertz (Hz), and intensity is measured in Decibels (dB). The human ear is capable of hearing sound over a range of frequencies from 20 (very low-pitched) to 20,000Hz (extremely high-pitched), but the most important frequencies for hearing speech are between 300 and 3,400Hz.

Because speech sounds vary in terms of pitch and loudness, some sounds are affected more than others by different degrees and types of hearing loss. For example, in the case of sensorineural hearing loss, there is typically more hearing loss in the higher frequencies, so people have more difficulty hearing high-pitched sounds like birds chirping, whispering, or speech sounds like *f, s,* and *th.* For hearing loss associated with fluid in the middle ear, the loss is more frequently in the lower frequencies (250 to 2,000 Hz), so depending on the degree of loss, vowels such as *a, e, i, o, u* and consonants such as *n, m, j, d, b,* and *g* may be harder to hear and discriminate.

Figure 4-2 shows familiar sounds and their pitch and loudness. Pitch is shown across the top—going from low-pitched sounds to high-pitched sounds. Loudness is shown along the side—going from the softest sound at the top to the loudest sound at the bottom.

Just to give you a reference point, normal conversation is typically around 60 dB in intensity, and whispering is around 30 dB. Children

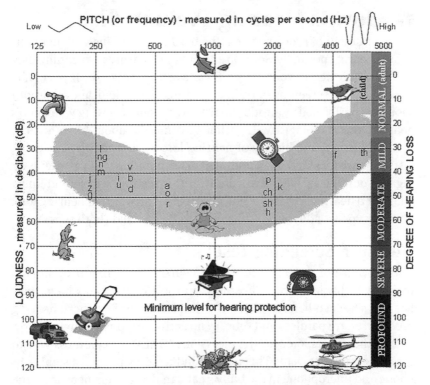

Fig. 4-2 © *The Alexander Bell Association. Reprinted by permission. Not to be reprinted without permission of the Alexander Bell Association.*

with mild hearing losses cannot distinguish sounds softer than 26–40 dB, so they have difficulty hearing speech that is soft or is far away. They may have difficulty hearing normal conversation if there is noise in the background. Children with moderate hearing loss cannot hear sounds softer than 41–55 dB) so they will have difficulty hearing speech that is spoken at a normal conversational level, even in a quiet room.

∷ Fluid in the Middle Ear and Hearing: A Chain Reaction

As the middle ear space changes from air-filled to fluid-filled, the fluid prevents the little bones and the eardrum from moving as they should. As a result, the sound becomes dampened and does not travel as easily to the inner ear.

∷ How Is Hearing Evaluated?

A number of procedures can be used to determine whether your baby is hearing normally. Some are screening measures—meaning they will tell you whether your baby *might* have a hearing loss. If your baby fails a hearing screening, a full hearing test (audiological evaluation) should be performed by an audiologist. In addition to testing your child's hearing, the audiologist will gather information about birth history, medical history, and history of hearing loss in your family. The exact tests that are included in an audiological evaluation will vary depending on your child's age. However, after this testing, you should know whether a hearing loss is present, the degree (amount) of hearing loss, and the type (conductive or sensorineural) or mixed (both types).

Newborn Screening Tests

Because of universal newborn hearing screening programs, a majority of babies born in hospitals in the United States have their hearing screened before leaving the hospital. These newborn hearing procedures are painless and require no active response from the baby. One of these tests, otoacoustic emissions (OAEs), is a painless way to assess hearing in a baby. This test is conducted by placing a small earphone and microphone in the baby's ear canal and then measuring the amount of sound echoing into the middle ear space in response to sound stimulating the cochlea. If no sound is measured in the middle ear, this may mean there is a problem with either the outer, middle, or inner ear.

Auditory brainstem response (ABR) is also used for newborn hearing screening or as part of a more in-depth audiological evaluation. ABR evaluates the inner ear or nerves associated with hearing. While the baby is sleeping, electrodes are placed on her head (and earphones on her ears), and recordings are taken of brainwave activity in response to sound. With ABR, it is possible to determine the quietest sound that the baby can hear across different frequencies.

It is not uncommon for a baby to fail her newborn hearing screening. Often this is because there is fluid in the middle ear cavity or other debris in the external ear canal, and often this blockage goes away a few days after birth. When a baby fails the newborn screening, she is rescreened before leaving the hospital or soon after. If she fails again, she will be referred for a more in-depth hearing test conducted by an audiologist who specializes in testing babies and young children.

Middle Ear Exams

If there are concerns about your baby's hearing, an audiologist can do a number of procedures that provide information about the middle ear, without actually requiring a response from your child. The first of these is *otoscopy,* which includes looking into your child's ear canal with an instrument called an otoscope. This allows the audiologist to see if there is redness, bubbles, a hole in the eardrum, possible fluid behind the eardrum, or even wax in the ear canal. The audiologist can also use *tympanometry,* a procedure in which air is pushed into the ear canal using a tiny rubber probe inserted into your child's ear. This measures how well the eardrum moves and can provide further verification of a hole in the eardrum, the status of ear tubes (see below), or whether there is negative or positive pressure in the middle ear space. Next, *acoustic reflex measures* provide information about whether the hearing loss is conductive or sensorineural based on how loud a sound needs to be to cause contraction of a tiny muscle in the middle ear.

All of these tests are quick and painless and can be easily performed at a cleft palate team visit or during an office visit to an audiologist. The information obtained from these tests can help the audiologist know whether to refer your child to her pediatrician or pediatric otolaryngologist (an ear, nose, and throat doctor or ENT) for medical management and can help to confirm the results of pure tone testing (described below).

Pure Tone Testing

Most adults are familiar with pure tone testing even if they don't know that that is what it is called. Through pure tone testing, the audiologist can tell what the quietest sound is that a person can hear at different frequencies or tones, from very low to very high. Earphones are placed over the ears, and the tones are sent to the earphones, first to one ear and then to the other. We raise our hand when we hear the sound, and the audiologist records our responses.

When testing a baby or child who is too young to raise her hand in response to sounds, visual reinforcement audiology (VRA) or conditioned play audiometry (CPA) can be used. With VRA (appropriate for a baby from six months to two years of age), the baby is trained to look at the source of the sound (for instance, toward a speaker to her right or left) by reinforcing her for correct looking each time the sound is presented. The reinforcement is visual and typically includes a light that flashes or an interesting toy that moves.

CPA is used for children between the ages of about two and five, and involves a conditioning procedure. With this procedure, the child is taught to do something (e.g., put a block in a pail) when she hears a sound. If the child will tolerate earphones, these tests will provide information about hearing in each ear separately and across all different frequencies and loudness levels. Otherwise, the test gives a general idea of how well the child is able to hear using both ears but will not tell you if there is a problem with hearing in one ear.

Finally, if there is some sort of blockage in the middle ear, pure tone bone conduction testing may be indicated. In order to go around the blockage, a small vibrator is placed behind the child's ear or on her forehead. The signals that are sent through the vibrator cause slight vibrations of the skull that go directly to the inner ear or cochlea (bypassing the outer and middle ears). This helps the audiologist determine if the problem identified is conductive or sensorineural.

■■ When Should Your Child's Hearing Be Tested?

If your baby is being followed by a cleft palate team, she should have her hearing tested as part of the team visit on at least a yearly basis. If your child fails a hearing test, ask your audiologist when you should schedule a follow-up hearing test to be sure that hearing has returned to normal. Additionally, if your child has had middle ear fluid that lasted for three months or more, be sure to ask the audiologist if a follow-up hearing assessment is needed. (See otitis media with effusion, above.) Finally, any time you think your baby is not hearing normally, you can contact the team audiologist and ask that a hearing test be scheduled.

According to the Centers for Disease Control and Prevention, signs that your baby or young child should have her hearing tested include the following:

- does not look at the sources of sound (after about six months) or "startle" at a loud sound;
- does not respond by turning her head when you call her name, but will do so when she sees you;
- responds to some sounds but not others;
- is not saying words by around one year or seems to be delayed in speech and language;
- does not follow directions.

▪▪ What Are the Signs of an Ear Infection?

In order to minimize the impact that ear infections have on hearing, ear disease must be identified and monitored both by your child's physician and by you, the parent. When your child is a baby and unable to tell you her ears hurt, it is up to you to recognize signs that she may have an infection. According to the Centers for Disease Control and Prevention, the following signs are associated with ear infections:

- excessive crying,
- drainage from the ear,
- fever,
- headache,
- problems sleeping, and
- problems with balance or hearing.

In its publication entitled *Causes of Hearing Loss in Children*, the American Speech-Language-Hearing Association (ASHA) identified six signs other than pain and fever that may indicate the presence of repeated episodes of fluid in the ear and possibly reduced hearing:

- inattentiveness,
- wanting the television or radio louder than usual,

- misunderstanding directions,
- listlessness,
- unexplained irritability,
- pulling or scratching at the ears.

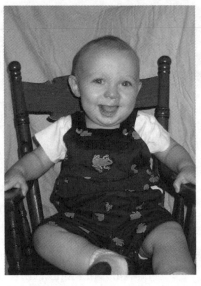

If you think your child has an ear infection, you should consult your physician as soon as possible to determine the best medical or surgical treatment. If left untreated, middle ear infections can rupture the eardrum. If your child experiences repeated ear infections, consult the audiologist on your child's cleft palate team to determine the severity of any accompanying hearing loss. In addition, an SLP can provide information about your child's speech and language performance and help you to identify appropriate therapy services when needed.

:: How Ear Infections Are Treated

As mentioned above, in some cases, ear infections clear up on their own, but if they do not, the most common treatment is antibiotics. For children with chronic or recurring ear infections, an ENT surgeon may suggest placing ear tubes or pressure equalization (PE) tubes in your child's eardrum so that that fluid can drain. Both of these treatments, along with research supporting their use, are described below.

Antibiotics

In the past, antibiotics were commonly used to treat AOM; however, physicians are becoming concerned about the overuse of these drugs. With time and repeated usage, the germs that are living in our bodies build up a resistance to the antibiotics. Then, the typical antibiotics are not strong enough to work on these more resistant germs. Researchers and physicians have been attempting to determine just how effective antibiotics are compared to a "wait-and-see" approach for the treatment of AOM.

A review of studies examining the effectiveness of antibiotics to treat OME in children was published in January 2013. The reviewers examined 12 studies involving a total of 3,317 children and concluded that antibiotics were not that effective in treating AOM when compared to a placebo treatment. They did not find that more children who were given antibiotics (compared to those who were not given antibiotics) were pain-free one day later, and only a few more children who were given antibiotics were pain-free a few days later. The children treated with antibiotics were also not found to have better hearing. That being said, those receiving antibiotics experienced fewer ear infections in the other ear and fewer perforated eardrums. The reviewers also added that antibiotics were more helpful for babies with AOM who were less than twenty-four months old and who had infection in both ears and discharge from the ears (Venekamp, Sanders, Glasziou, Del Mar, & Rovers, 2013).

Reports like these have prompted some doctors to wait and prescribe antibiotics only if the symptoms continue or become worse after a few days (typically forty-eight to seventy-two hours).

The American Academy of Pediatrics and American Academy of Family Physicians have published guidelines for treatment of AOM in young children, addressing the issue of whether it is better to wait and see or prescribe antibiotics. The first committee of experts met in 2000 and reviewed the same body of research described above. The guidelines were published in the journal *Pediatrics* in 2004. In 2009, a new committee was convened to reconsider the current guidelines and review any new research published since the previous review. This document was published in the journal *Pediatrics* in 2013. The committee concluded that a number of factors have to be considered when choosing between prescribing antibiotics and the wait-and-see approach. These include the age of the child, how sick the child is, how certain the physician is about the diagnosis of AOM, and the options for reevaluation and access to medication, if needed. For example, the guidelines suggest that antibiotics be prescribed for children under two years of age with bilateral AOM even if they don't appear to have high fever or pain.

For you as parents of a child with CP, it is important to understand that the guidelines for treating ear infections were developed for an "otherwise healthy child without underlying conditions that may alter the natural course of AOM, including but not limited to...the cleft palate" (Lieberthal, et al., 2013, p. e966). Your child's doctors may not

:: How to Find Out about Best Practices for Different Medical Conditions

For unbiased reviews of the research that is available on treatments for many health-related conditions, a good place to go is the Cochrane Reviews (http://www.cochrane.org/ cochrane-reviews). There, reviews are compiled by an international, not-for profit organization called the Cochrane Collaboration (http:// www.cochrane.org). The reviews are carried out by experts in a specific area and are based on the most current research. Once a question is identified (e.g., Do ear tubes decrease the frequency of ear infections in children?), a group of researchers review all the studies on the topic. Based on the available information, they come up with a decision about whether or not the treatment works. Sometimes there is strong evidence either for or against a certain treatment. For other treatments, there may not be enough research (or well-designed research) to draw a conclusion, and reviewers will tell you that as well. As new information becomes available, the reviews are revised and updated.

A similar website designed as a resource for learning about the latest research for different medical conditions is hosted by the Agency for Healthcare Research and Quality (http://www.ahrq. gov/index.html). One of the many resources on this website is the National Guidelines Clearinghouse (http://www.guideline.gov), which houses clinical practice guidelines (including the complete guidelines for management of AOE) for over two thousand medical conditions, treatments, and other health-related services.

necessarily follow these guidelines when deciding whether to prescribe antibiotics for ear infections. But treatment will likely depend on many factors, such as your child's age, overall health status, frequency of ear infections, and other considerations. Of course, you will want to contact your child's physician if you suspect your child has an ear infection to determine the best course of action.

Ear Tubes

Another popular approach to treatment of ear infections is *myringotomy* (a small incision) with insertion of ear tubes in the eardrum.

According to the American Academy of Otolaryngology-Head and Neck Surgery, myringotomy is the most common surgery requiring anesthesia performed on young children. More than 500,000 children undergo this procedure every year.

These tubes have many different names: myringotomy tubes, pressure equalization tubes, tympanostomy tubes, ventilation tubes, grommets, etc. They are small plastic, metal, or Teflon tubes that are designed to let air into the middle ear so that fluid does not build up and cause ear infections and hearing loss (see Figure 4-3). Insertion of the ear tubes may be scheduled at the time of another surgery (e.g., lip repair or palate repair). The tubes may stay in for six to twelve months or longer. They typically fall out themselves, and the hole in the eardrum closes as it heals.

Because of the high rate of ear infections in babies and young children with CP, some teams believe in aggressive otologic (ear) management. This typically means that tubes are placed at the time of lip repair or palate repair (for babies with cleft palate only) and are replaced if they come out or become blocked. More recently, some physicians have become more cautious, as it has been noted that multiple tube insertions may cause permanent damage to the eardrum.

A number of research studies have been carried out to determine if early tube placement for babies with CP improves hearing or has other positive or negative effects on the health of the middle ear, speech and language development, or quality of life. A review of thirty-three of these studies was published in the *Cleft Palate-Craniofacial Journal* in 2009. Some of the studies found that early tube placement resulted in more improvements in children's speech, language, or hearing status and number of ear infections, at least in the short term. Others found that there were no

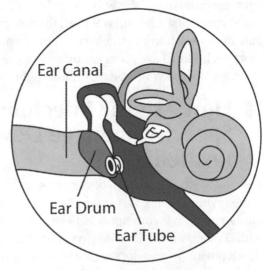

Fig. 4-3 *Ear Tube.*

differences between the children with and without tubes, and some reported complications (e.g., scarring of the eardrum, permanent perforations in the eardrum, etc.) associated with tube placement in younger children. Because of the disagreements across studies, the authors concluded that we do not know if tubes are beneficial and that more study is needed (Ponduri, Bradley, Ellis, Brookes, Sandy, & Ness, 2009).

When we consulted the Cochrane Reviews concerning use of ear tubes for treatment of otitis media, we found no reviews on the effectiveness of ear tubes for children with CP. However, there were reviews for children without CP who were typically otherwise healthy. A review focusing on children under three year of age with AOM concluded that children with ear tubes were more likely to have either fewer or no new episodes of AOM in the first six months after placement of the tubes (McDonald, Langton Hewer, & Nunez, 2008). The reviewers also concluded that ear tubes improved hearing in the first six months but not for the long term. However, they did not note any difference in language skills for children who had tubes placed. It is important to note that the reviewers made the disclaimer that none of these studies included children already showing speech and language delays or other conditions associated with a higher occurrence of ear infections such as CP.

The reviewers commented that some subgroups of children, including those that attend daycare, benefit more from ear tubes (Browning, Rovers, Williamson, & Burton, 2010). If your baby suffers from ear infections, she will likely be under the care of a pediatric otolaryngologist who will weigh all the potential positive and negative outcomes to determine the best treatment options. The good news is that the children have fewer ear infections the older they get, with most children "outgrowing" them by about eight to ten years of age.

▪ How Are Ear Infections and Speech-Language Development Related?

As SLPs, our major concern is how ear infections and the accompanying hearing loss influence your child's speech and language development. It is commonly believed that the hearing loss associated with OME may result in delays in young children's speech and language development. In an effort to prove or refute this proposal, over a hundred studies have been carried out over a period of more than forty years (Roberts, Rosenfeld, & Ziesel, 2004). A synthesis of research on this topic, which was published in the journal *Pediatrics* in 2004, concluded that for children who are "otherwise healthy," OME either has no impact on later speech and language development or a very small impact (Roberts, Rosenfeld, & Ziesel, 2004). However, that does not mean that for any individual child or for your child, OME would not have a significant impact.

You are probably wondering if researchers have attempted to look at this relationship in children with CP. Yes, a few have. A review of those studies concluded that an association between OME and later speech and language abilities exists, but the evidence for a direct causal relationship is just not there. That is, we cannot say that OME is the cause of speech and language delays for children with CP.

In our own research, we evaluated the speech and language skills of a group of children with CP from the time they were six months of age until they were thirty-nine months of age or older. When we looked at their speech and language skills and their history of ear infections and hearing levels, we found that there were children who had many episodes of OME with normal speech and language development and others who had no or very few episodes of OME with delayed speech and language development.

It is difficult to say for any individual child with CP exactly what may be contributing to any delays that may occur. We want to make sure that every child with CP has the optimal environment for speech and language learning. Such an environment includes monitoring ear infections, hearing status, and speech and language development. The professionals with expertise in these areas, including your child's physician, audiologist, and SLP, will be able to advise you about your child's status in all of these areas and the best course of treatment. If your child has repeated ear infections, you and the professionals working with your child will need to balance the risks that may be associated with more aggressive treatment against the risk of speech and language delay that may result from repeated ear infections and associated hearing loss.

Of course, the optimal environment for speech and language learning does not just include monitoring and treating medical conditions. It also includes plentiful support and practice with communication skills provided by parents, SLPs, and others, as described in Chapter 6.

■■ How Can You Reduce or Lessen the Impact of Ear Infections and Reduced Hearing?

While you cannot control most of the factors that put your baby at risk for ear infections, you can take steps that may reduce their occurrence or make modifications in your environment that may lessen the impact. We would like to begin with these recommendations from the Centers for Disease Control and Prevention and the National Institutes of Health–National Institute on Deafness and Other Communication Disorders that might help to prevent ear infections in your baby or young child:

1. Avoid exposure to pollutants such as cigarette smoke or pollution from the air.
2. Vaccinate your child against the flu and with the 13-valent pneumococcal conjugate vaccine (PCV13). Make sure that other vaccinations for your child and family members are also current.
3. Nurse your baby in an upright position, and if possible, nurse or provide your baby with breast milk for up to twelve months.
4. Avoid exposing your child to other sick children.

Another important thing that you can do is to take the appropriate action when you suspect that your baby has an ear infection or has reduced hearing. In the section above, we described characteristics that should alert you that something might be wrong. As we mentioned previously, parents are often unaware that their young child has OME until it is diagnosed by a physician or identified during hearing testing. However, we have often wondered if young children with chronic infections and good speech and language skills do so well because their parents are more aware of the signs/symptoms and seek medical interventions and compensate for times when hearing may not be optimal by providing extra language stimulation.

A publication of the National Center for Early Development and Learning and the American Speech-Language-Hearing Association (ASHA) offers information for families and professionals who are dealing with babies and young children who experience frequent ear infections. They have provided a list of things that you can do with your child that will hopefully lessen the impact of ear infections on speech and language development:

- Be sure that you have your child's attention before speaking.
- Be sure your child is close to whoever is speaking (within three feet).
- Be sure that your child can see your face. Speak naturally and normally, but repeat important words.
- Consider adding pictures or gestures when you talk.
- Check that your child understands what you are saying by asking her questions.
- Decrease distractions that make it harder for her to hear, especially background noise (e.g., television, noisy appliances, and toys).

We would like to add to this list that you should take advantage of naturally occurring activities throughout the day to stimulate your child's speech and language development. We refer you to the activities described in Chapter 7 and suggest you incorporate the steps above when interacting with your child.

▪▪ Summary

Young children with cleft palate are at risk for middle ear problems and associated hearing loss, especially during the early years. There is some controversy about the best way to treat middle ear disease in all children, including those with CP. Although all professionals rely on research to guide their practice, it is important to remember that the studies describe average performance, and that in all these studies, there are individual children who do better than the average child and others who do worse than the average child with the treatments described. Careful monitoring of your child's middle ear status, hearing, and speech and language development is imperative to lessen the potential impact of middle ear disease on her development.

5

SURGERY
AND
DENTAL CARE

Like most parents, you probably have some concerns about the surgery that will be needed to correct your baby's cleft lip and palate (CLP). And although you are probably anxious for the cleft to be repaired, you may be concerned about your child going under anesthesia at such a young age and have a lot of questions about what will happen during and after the surgery. How many surgeries will your child require? What is the recovery process like? What can you do to prepare your child for the experience?

If you have spent time talking to parents of other children with clefts and have read a lot about the condition and its treatment, you may also be wondering why your surgeon's plan for your child is different from others you have heard about. These are commonly asked questions, and your surgeon will discuss them with you at length.

The good news is that because CLP is among the most common congenital problems affecting young children, a lot of attention has been given to learning how to treat it. Thanks to advances in treatment, cosmetic and speech outcomes are better than ever.

Because each child's cleft condition is somewhat different, the exact procedures performed and the timetable for different procedures is not always the same. Our goal in this chapter is to provide you with an overview of the different operations and dental treatments that are commonly used in children with cleft lip and palate. Because we are not surgeons or dental specialists and because we do not have personal knowledge of your child, we may not answer all of the questions that you have. Hopefully, though, the information provided here will help you frame the questions that you want to ask.

As the time of your child's first surgery approaches, we would encourage you to begin keeping a diary. Write down all of the questions that come to mind so that you can have an informative conversation with your child's surgeon. Writing down your questions and recording the responses you receive is very important. There will be times when your child is being seen by multiple specialists on the cleft palate team, and it will become difficult to remember all of the information you have been provided. Once you get into the routine of keeping a diary, we think you will be glad you did. The questions and answers that you record will form a story that you will be able to share with your child as he gets older and begins asking questions about his condition and how it was treated. Ultimately, that story may provide the foundation for your child's responses to questions that his peers may ask when he is older.

The types of operations that are used to repair a cleft lip and a cleft palate differ considerably among surgeons. So too does the age of the child at the time of each operation. The information below is provided as a general overview of surgical management and may or may not reflect the plan that your child's surgeon has in mind. The decisions that your child's surgeon makes about when and how to repair the cleft may be influenced by a number of factors. These include (but are not limited to) the following:

1. your child's general health,
2. the severity of the cleft,
3. the surgeon's personal preferences.

This chapter also covers some issues related to dental care that are specific to children with CLP.

▐▌ Cleft Lip Surgery

If your baby has both a cleft lip (CL) and cleft palate (CP), the lip is usually repaired first. Surgery to repair a cleft lip is performed for most babies in the United States when they are approximately two to four months old. The goals of surgery are both esthetic and functional: the lip should look as normal as possible at rest and during facial animation, speaking, and eating.

Cleft lip surgery involves repairing the circular lip muscle (*orbicularis oris*), creating the cupid's bow, and making the upper lip and base of the nose symmetrical—all with minimal scarring. These goals are more easily accomplished in some children than others. Although a surgeon's skill is an important factor in any surgical outcome, it is important to recognize that the size of the original cleft (the amount of missing tissue) plays a large role in determining how well the goals of the surgery are met.

Cleft lip repair may be more difficult if there is a wide cleft lip with a large gap in the gum (*alveolus*) and, often, if the central portion of the upper jaw (*premaxilla*) protrudes. Several options are available to reduce the cleft gap and the premaxilla protrusion:

1. The surgeon might ask you to tape your baby's lip for a while prior to surgery. Surgical tape placed across the cleft will bring the two sides of the lip closer together in a more natural position. This will narrow the cleft and result in less tension on the stitches following surgery. Taping may be done with or without an intraoral appliance (see the Presurgical Orthopedic Therapy section below).

2. The surgeon may perform a preliminary lip closure with muscle repair (called a lip adhesion) first. Then, a number of months later, he or she performs a definitive lip repair, to make the lip look as normal as possible.

When a cleft occurs on each side of the mouth (bilateral cleft lip), some surgeons repair both sides at once, while others prefer to repair one side first, then the other side in a separate operation some time later.

A number of different operations are used to repair a cleft lip, and it is beyond the scope of this book to describe them in detail. In a typical surgical repair, incisions are made on either side of the cleft, resulting in flaps of tissue that are then joined with sutures (stitches) to close the cleft. The operation, which includes initial repair of the nose as well, usually lasts approximately two to four hours (for unilateral CL, two to three hours; for bilateral CL, three to four hours) and is performed under general anesthesia. Babies are usually admitted to the hospital overnight, but sometimes a longer stay is needed.

Your child's lip scar will be red and stiff following the surgery and will remain so for several months. Over time, you will notice that the redness will fade and the scar will soften. Like other parents, you probably wonder whether there is there anything you can do to improve the appearance of the scar. For instance, do vitamins, lotions, and scar creams help the appearance of scars? Will lip massage help soften a rigid scar? These questions receive quite a bit of attention on the Internet, but to our knowledge there is no definitive answer. As pointed out by the Cleft Palate Foundation in its fact sheet, *Answers to Common Questions about Scars*, "There is no consistent evidence" that vitamin E, aloe vera, and cocoa butter "improve the long-term appearance" of a scar.

Although we are all tempted from time to time to seek out answers to questions on the Internet, it is important to remember that manufacturers of products and authors of publications do not know your child or his specific needs. When you are in doubt about how to proceed, your child's physician is your best source for answers regarding your child's surgery and the long-term outcomes associated with it.

Although cleft lip surgery leaves a permanent visible scar, "touch-up" surgery may be done to improve the appearance, and sometimes function, of the lip (and/or nose) as the child grows. This is often done at the same time as another operation to minimize the number of anesthesias for the child and disruptions for the family.

Considerations Prior to Surgery

In their publication entitled *Cleft Surgery*, the Cleft Palate Foundation lists the following questions you may want to ask your surgeon prior to your baby's surgery:

1. How old does my child have to be for this surgery? Why?
2. How long will my child have to be in the hospital?
3. Can more than one procedure be performed during the same operation?
4. How do I feed my baby after repair?
5. How can I manage any pain or discomfort that my child experiences?
6. How long should I plan to take off from work to care for my child?
7. How many hours will my child be under anesthesia?
8. How will my child behave after surgery?

9. What problems should I watch for after my child comes home from the hospital?

Having answers to each of these questions before your child's surgery will ensure that you know what to expect during and after the surgery and can plan accordingly.

Your Child's Needs Following Surgery

There is a lot of information on the Internet about postoperative lip and palate care. If you frequently seek out information on the Internet, be aware that your surgeon's philosophy about the care your child needs following surgery (including pain management and feeding) may not be the same as another surgeon's. Before discharging your child from the hospital following lip surgery, your child's surgeon will probably discuss with you the importance of keeping the suture site clean to prevent infection. Some surgeons ask parents to clean the stitches and surrounding area several times a day, while others prefer that the incision site be left alone. If your child's surgeon wants you to clean the incision, he or she will give you specific instructions for how to do that and what to use.

Some surgeons (but not all) place padded arm restraints on a baby's arms after lip surgery. This prevents the baby from bending his elbows and bringing his hands or other hard objects to his mouth. If your baby has arm restraints, the surgeon will probably recommend that you remove them for short periods of time (five to fifteen minutes) throughout the day in order to "exercise" the arm. Your baby must be carefully supervised during this time to ensure that he does not put his fingers (or anything else) in his mouth.

As explained in Chapter 3, your surgeon will provide you with special instructions for feeding your child following lip surgery. Although many surgeons permit feeding from a bottle or breast in the immediate postoperative period, some recommend the use of particular feeders (such as syringe feeders) for a week or longer following surgery. This is to ensure that the stitches are not damaged by an object placed in the mouth or the tension associated with sucking. Pacifiers are usually not permitted at all for the same reason. It is important that you follow your surgeon's instructions very closely in order to avoid injury and promote healing of the surgical site.

Your child will probably be given pain medication while he is in the hospital. On discharge, some surgeons recommend prescription-strength pain medication, while others recommend over-the-counter medications if needed. If your child is irritable and fussy, comfort him with cuddling and rocking. Remember, he has a lot to be fussy about! In addition to any soreness that may be present, he has lost familiar items that have brought him comfort in the past (bottle and pacifier). The loss of those items, along with the movement restrictions that arm restraints impose, can frustrate a baby and lead to fussiness. Your baby will rely on you during this time for comfort and distraction.

▪▪ Cleft Palate Surgery

In the United States, cleft palate surgery is usually performed when the child is between ten to twelve months of age. Most surgeons perform a one-stage repair, meaning both the hard and soft palate are repaired at the same time. Although most surgeons prefer to close the palate prior to a baby's first birthday to ensure that the baby has an intact palate as speech develops, surgery may be modified or delayed when the cleft is large or there are complicating medical issues such as an unstable upper airway or congenital heart disease.

Some surgeons choose to delay surgery on the hard palate in the hope of minimizing negative effects of palate surgery on growth of the bones of the midface. In such cases, a two-stage repair is performed with the soft palate repaired prior to a child's first birthday and the hard palate closed at a later time. When closure of the hard palate cleft is delayed, many centers cover the remaining hard palate cleft with a custom plastic appliance (obturator), similar to an orthodontic retainer, until the cleft is surgically repaired. This device prevents loss of air through the cleft into the nose during speech production and minimizes nasal regurgitation with eating. One-stage cleft palate repairs are far more common in the United States than two-stage repairs.

The primary goal of palatal surgery is to create an intact palate that will separate the nose from the mouth and function appropriately for normal speech and swallowing. Anecdotal reports from professionals suggest that other potential benefits of palatal surgery may include fewer upper respiratory infections and ear infections. Evidence to support these potential benefits is needed, however.

Types of Operations

The type of palatal operation that is performed on your child will depend upon the size of the cleft, the amount of tissue available next to the cleft, and your surgeon's preference. Regardless of which specific operation your surgeon uses, the actual surgery will *not* involve moving the palatal bones together to cover the cleft. In most cases, the tissue (skin) that covers the bone next to each side of the cleft is partially separated from the bone, moved over the cleft, and sutured together.

Hard palate clefts are typically repaired using a two-layer closure technique. Flaps of nasal tissue are used to close the floor of the nose, while flaps of oral tissue next to the cleft are used to close the oral surface of the cleft. A diagram of a simple palatal repair is shown in Figure 5-1 (a-d). The dotted lines in Figure 5-1a represent the incisions that are made through the palatal tissue to the bone. Figure 5-1b depicts the tissue flaps that are released when the incisions are made. The nasal surface of the palate has been closed in Figure 5-1c, and the oral surface of the palate is closed in Figure 5-1d. Note that the elongated white areas on either side of the palate in Figures 5-1c and 5-1d represent the areas of bone from which the flaps were moved. These areas are raw immediately after surgery, but heal within a week or two.

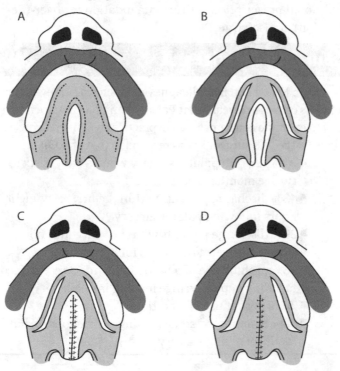

Fig. 5-1 *Simple Palate Repair.*

The soft palate contains a muscle that is critical for *velopharyngeal closure*. Recall that velopharyngeal closure* refers to the ability of the soft palate to move back and up against the back wall of the throat to close off the nose during speech. This movement is accomplished largely through the contraction of a muscle in the soft palate known as the *levator veli palatini* muscle. Most surgeons connect the two congenitally separated right and left halves of this muscle at the time that they repair the soft palate to optimize palatal motion following surgery. That procedure is known as an *intravelar veloplasty*.

Surgical repair of a CP usually takes approximately two hours (sometimes longer), and you can expect your child to be hospitalized for one to two days. Your child will have stitches in the roof of his mouth following surgery. Frequently, the stitches that are used dissolve on their own and do not need to be removed. Your child's surgeon will let you know the type of stitches that your child has and whether they must be removed. Your child will be given pain medication in the hospital to help with the soreness, and you may be provided with an additional prescription (or recommendation for over-the-counter medication) at discharge.

∷ Surgical Practices

Evan Katzel and his colleagues conducted a survey of surgeon members of the American Cleft Palate-Craniofacial Association in 2009 to examine common surgical practices when repairing a cleft palate. Of the 288 surgeons who responded (out of 803):

- 74% perform palatal surgery when a baby is six to twelve months of age.
- 43% discharge patients within the first forty-eight hours following palatal surgery.
- 39% discharge patients within twenty-four hours.
- 85% require arm restraints following surgery.
- 33% prohibit use of a bottle following surgery, recommending cup or syringe feeding instead.
- 58% permit use of a bottle.
- 98% recommend some feeding restrictions on hard foods following surgery.

---

* *"Velo" in the word velopharyngeal refers to the "velum" or soft palate. "Pharyngeal" refers to the throat.*

Some surgeons permit the use of some types of bottles following palatal surgery, but others recommend feeding with a cup and advise against the use of bottles, sippy cups with spouts or straws, and pacifiers to ensure that the incision site heals without risk of trauma to the stitches. A liquid diet and soft foods will typically be recommended for a period of up to two weeks (sometimes longer). Arm restraints may once again be placed on your child's arms to ensure that he cannot bend his elbows and bring his hands (or anything else) to his mouth. If your surgeon recommends arm restraints, they will probably be kept in place for a couple of weeks as the palate heals.

As is true following lip surgery, your child will depend on you for comfort throughout his hospitalization. Remember, he will most likely be a baby if a one-stage operation is performed. But if a two-stage operation is performed, the soft palate may be repaired when he is less than a year old, but the hard palate may not be repaired until he is a toddler or preschooler. Since hospitals are rarely found on an adult's list of favorite places to go, it should come as no surprise that preschoolers and older children also may find the environment confusing and scary at times. Between strangers walking in and out of the room, discomfort associated with the incision site, and movement restrictions that are imposed by arm restraints (if they are used), your child may be very irritable at times.

It is a good idea to bring along a few of your child's comfort items, such as favorite toys, books, and videos, so that you can distract him when necessary. If he is an older toddler or preschooler, you may also want to prepare him for the hospital by describing what will happen in very general terms. Although children do not need a lot of detail, they do need to know the basic steps of what will happen when they arrive at the hospital. A very brief description might sound something like this:

"We will wake up very early tomorrow and go to the hospital so they can fix the hole in your mouth. You will not be able to eat breakfast before we go. When we get to the hospital, a nurse will give you some pajamas to put on and then may give you some medicine to drink that will make you sleepy. I will wait with you until the doctor comes to take you to a special room, called an operating room. That's where they will fix your mouth. I can't go with you but will wait right outside the room. The doctor (or nurse) will take you to the operating room and give you some

*more medicine that will make you sleep. You will be asleep while
they are fixing your mouth. Once the doctor has finished, they
will wake you up. I will be there when you wake up. The inside of
your mouth will be sore for a few days, but the doctor will give you
some medicine to make it feel better. You will have to stay in the
hospital for a day or two while your mouth gets better and I will be
right there with you. Let's think of some movies, books, and toys
you can take with you."*

A number of children's books have been written to describe what
happens in a hospital (such as *Franklin Goes to the Hospital* and *Little
Critter: My Trip to the Hospital*). You may want to have one of these
books on hand when you talk to your child about going to the hospital.

Palatal Fistula

One possible complication of palatal surgery is the development of
a hole in the palate connecting the mouth and nose. This hole, known as
a *palatal fistula*, may occur due to disruption of the surgical site, usually
due to excessive tension on the repair site or poor blood supply. A fistula
may also result from incomplete closure of the cleft palate (due to the
type of operation or the size of the cleft or its configuration). Fistulas
due to repair breakdown occur most commonly at the junction of the
hard and soft palates; fistulas due to nonrepair usually are in the front
of the hard palate, in the gum ridge (*alveolus*), or both. The size of a
palatal fistula varies considerably, ranging from breakdown of a large
portion of the repair (essentially reopening the cleft) to a hole no larger
than a pinpoint. Your child's surgeon will check for a fistula when he
is seen for follow-up in the weeks after surgery and in subsequent cleft
palate team visits.

The presence of a small palatal fistula in and of itself is of little
concern. Because palatal repairs are performed in two layers, a "hole"
that is seen on the hard palate may not always be open into the nose.
And even when a fistula is open, it may not be associated with any
obvious symptoms. A palatal fistula is of concern when it results in
liquids and food passing into the nose during eating and/or air passing
into the nose during speech. If your child has *audible nasal emission*
(snorting), the speech-language pathologist on your cleft palate team
can help determine whether the air passing through your child's nose is
the result of a palatal fistula or an inability to achieve velopharyngeal

closure (known as *velopharyngeal inadequacy* = VPI). When closure of the fistula is needed, it can be repaired surgically or covered (obturated) using a dental appliance.

Success Rate of Palatal Surgery

As mentioned above, the primary goal of palatal surgery is to close the cleft and create a soft palate that is capable of separating the mouth and nose during speech (defined earlier as velopharyngeal closure). Consequently, the success of the surgery is usually measured in terms of the percentage of children who achieve adequate velopharyngeal closure for speech. It is reported that about 75 to 80 percent of all children who have their CP repaired are able to achieve adequate velopharyngeal closure following surgery. The remaining 20 to 25 percent have difficulty achieving velopharyngeal closure. This percentage varies considerably across surgeons and depends on a number of factors, including the surgeon's skill, the type of procedure used, and the severity of the cleft.

Children who have difficulty with velopharyngeal closure may have speech that sounds excessively nasal (hypernasal). When hypernasality (too much air resonating in the nose) is severe enough to call attention to a child's speech or prevent him from being understood, additional surgery is typically recommended. The speech-language pathologist on your child's cleft palate team will monitor your child's speech closely for several years following the initial palatal surgery to look for signs of VPI. It is important to point out that even when VPI is suspected in a very young child, the cleft palate team may decide to delay treatment until the child is old enough to tolerate the procedures used to study the velopharyngeal mechanism. See Chapter 8 for further discussion of this topic.

▪▪ Surgery for VPI

The primary reason to perform surgery for VPI is to improve nasal-sounding speech. Normal speech production is a dynamic process that requires air to flow into the nose for nasal consonants *(m, n, ng)* and into the mouth for all other speech sounds. To achieve the goal of normal speech, it is important for the surgeon to tailor the surgery to the child's anatomy and take advantage of the movement that is available when possible.

There are two operations that are routinely used in the United States and elsewhere to treat VPI: the *pharyngeal flap* and the *sphincter pharyngoplasty*. Both procedures are designed to make the opening from the throat into the back of the nose smaller so that the movement of the soft palate and the sides of the throat will be sufficient to close off the smaller hole(s). A third procedure, *pharyngeal augmentation,* is less commonly used but will be described below since it is an option for some patients. The fourth procedure, known as *palatal lengthening,* is an operation designed to lengthen the soft palate and reposition the muscle within it.

Keep in mind that some surgeons use only one of the procedures described below for all of their patients, but others may selectively use different procedures with different children depending on the specific problem that is present. For some children, nonsurgical management with a speech prosthesis (like an orthodontic retainer with an extension toward the back of the throat) is preferred due to concerns about obstructive sleep apnea or complicating medical conditions that make surgery more dangerous.

Pharyngeal Flap

The pharyngeal flap procedure (shown in Figure 5-2) involves taking tissue from the back wall of the throat and attaching it to the soft palate. This flap, which creates a permanent tissue bridge between the throat and the soft palate, covers most of the opening into the back of the nose, leaving two small openings (ports) on either side of the flap to allow air to move into the nose for nasal breathing. These openings also allow air to pass into the nose for production of nasal consonants during speech. Children who have good inward movement of the side walls of the throat are considered to be ideal candidates for this procedure since that movement is required to close off the openings on either side of the flap for all other speech sounds.

This operation usually lasts approximately an hour and a half and involves an overnight stay in the hospital (sometimes longer). Your child's throat will be sore following this procedure, and he may complain of a sore neck. A soft diet will be recommended for a period of time. Swelling around the incisions can result in nasal blockage, but that should get better with time. Because a large portion of the opening into the nose is covered by the flap, children often breathe through their mouth following this surgery, even once swelling subsides. You may be

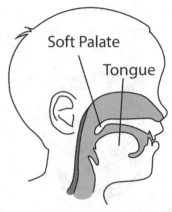
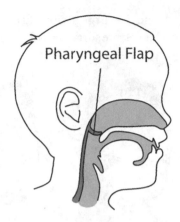

Fig. 5-2 *Pharyngeal flap.*

able to see the stitches along the roof of your child's mouth following this surgery, but you will typically not see the pharyngeal flap (it is higher in the throat).

Because of the swelling around the surgical site, your child may initially sound as if he has a bad cold when he talks. This type of speech resonance is known as *hyponasality* and occurs when you do not have enough air resonating in the nose. As the swelling goes down over a period of several months, the hyponasality should diminish and your child's resonance should sound increasingly normal.

Sphincter Pharyngoplasty

The sphincter pharyngoplasty* is a procedure that involves taking tissue flaps (muscular flaps) from either side of the mouth (behind the tonsils), bringing the ends together, and attaching them to the back of the throat. This permanently narrows the space between the nose and the mouth at the site of velopharyngeal closure, leaving a small central opening (port). (See Figure 5-3.) This operation brings the back of the throat as well as the side walls of the throat closer to the soft palate so that the palate does not have to move as far to close off the nose. Children who have short but mobile soft palates are considered to be good candidates for this procedure.

A sphincter pharyngoplasty usually takes about an hour and a half and typically involves an overnight stay in the hospital. Your child's throat will be sore following the procedure, and postoperative swelling

---

* *Pharyngoplasty is a term that simply refers to surgery in the throat.*

around the surgical site will probably result in hyponasality for a period of time. Some surgeons will recommend a soft diet following the surgery.

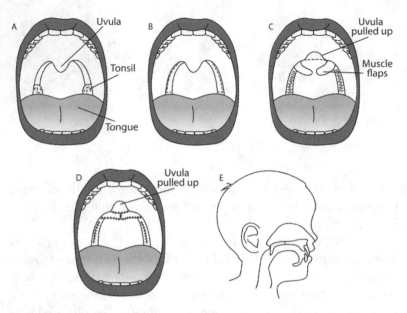

Fig. 5-3 *Sphincter Pharyngoplasty.*

Pharyngeal Augmentation

Pharyngeal augmentation is a less commonly performed procedure that is used in some centers. This procedure involves injecting or implanting a material (such as collagen, fat, or artificial materials) into the back wall of the throat at the level of velopharyngeal closure. The objective of the procedure is to create a bulge in the back wall of the throat, narrowing the distance that the palate must move to achieve velopharyngeal closure. (See Figure 5-4.)

Ideal candidates for this procedure are children who have small velo-

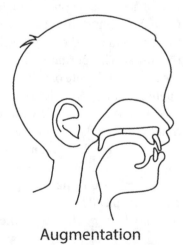

Augmentation

Fig. 5-4 *Pharyngeal Augmentation*

pharyngeal openings. Success of the procedure depends upon inserting the material at the precise location where the soft palate elevates. In some cases, the procedure must be repeated to achieve the expected results. Absorption, shrinkage, and migration of the material are infrequent complications that can occur with pharyngeal augmentation.

The pharyngeal augmentation procedure usually lasts about an hour. Your child may complain of a sore throat and stiff neck following this procedure. Unlike other procedures performed for VPI, which usually require an overnight stay in the hospital, this procedure is performed at some centers on an outpatient basis.

Palatal Lengthening

Palatal lengthening is a procedure that is typically performed when a child has a small velopharyngeal opening. The operation involves re-repairing the soft palate to lengthen it. In addition, the primary muscle that moves the soft palate is repositioned so that the soft palate moves better. By lengthening the soft palate and increasing its mobility, a child is now able to move the palate against the back wall of the throat to achieve velopharyngeal closure.

This operation usually lasts an hour and a half and involves an overnight stay in the hospital (sometimes longer). Your child's mouth will be sore following surgery and a soft diet will be recommended for a period of time.

Surgical Outcomes

It is important for you to know that for some children, neither the palate nor the side walls of the throat move much at all. For these children, the surgery that is performed will likely make the opening of the throat into the nose smaller, but speech still may not sound totally normal. Remember that speech is dynamic—sometimes we need air moving into the nose for nasal consonants, and sometimes we need all air moving into the mouth for other speech sounds. If a child's soft palate and walls of the throat do not move to open and close off the nose from the throat, it will be difficult for the surgeon to provide the child with a velopharyngeal mechanism that results in totally normal speech. The child's speech will probably sound much better following surgery, but he may still have some mild hypernasality or mild hyponasality.

The overall success rate of surgery for VPI is variable. In general, roughly 80 percent of children who receive this surgery can be expected to have normal resonance (that is, air is passing into and resonating in the mouth and nose at appropriate times). When the surgery "fails," most children still sound much better than they did prior to the surgery—they simply have speech that is slightly hypernasal or hyponasal.

▪▪ Bone Grafting

A complete cleft of the lip and palate typically extends through the lip, gum (alveolar) ridge, and palate (see Chapter 1). Although the lip and palate will typically be repaired in the child's first year of life, repair of the alveolar ridge will usually be delayed until he is older (to avoid interference with growth of the upper jaw). In this surgery, bone is taken from another part of the body. Usually, a small incision is made in the hip bone, and a portion of the soft, inner bone is removed. This bone is then added to the alveolar ridge in the cleft site. In addition, the surgeon repairs any residual opening into the nose, the palate (alveolar-nasal fistula), or both. The surgery is performed under anesthesia and usually takes approximately two hours. Your child will stay in the hospital overnight (sometimes longer) and will initially be on a liquid diet. Your child's surgeon will let you know when he can transition to a soft food diet and when he can resume contact sports and other physical activities.

Alveolar bone grafting is usually performed when a child is roughly eight to ten years of age, before his permanent canine teeth have erupted (when a child has a bilateral CLP, some surgeons prefer to repair each side at a different time). It provides stability of the dental arch (upper jaw that houses teeth), additional support for the base of the nose, and bony support for teeth surrounding the cleft. Many surgeons will take advantage of the general anesthesia necessary for alveolar bone grafting to perform a touch-up procedure on the lip or nose at the same time.

▪▪ Dental Management

Children with CP are at increased risk for cavities and tooth irregularities (missing or extra teeth), so your child should be routinely evaluated by a dentist. Some children with cleft palate need specialized dental care, particularly if they were born with a cleft that extends through the gum ridge. In this case, the stability of the dental arch has been disrupted, which can lead to arch collapse.

When a child has a unilateral CLP, the cleft side of the palate may collapse over time and move out of alignment with the rest of the dental arch.

When a child has a bilateral CLP, the central portion of the dental arch in the front of the mouth (*premaxilla*) is not attached to the palatal segments on either side. This usually results in the premaxilla rotating out of its proper position. Over time, the dental arches on either side may collapse and "lock out" the premaxilla. (See Figure 5-5.) This situation can complicate surgery for the lip and palate and lead to problems with the alignment of the upper and lower jaws as well as that of individual teeth.

How these problems are treated differs among cleft palate centers. Some cleft palate teams use procedures in infancy to either prevent the dental arch collapse or mold the palatal segments into their appropriate position prior to palatal surgery. Others treat the problem when the child is older.

Although cleft palate teams may use different approaches to treat the problems associated with cleft lip and palate, their long-term goals are the same. Research is currently underway to examine the long-term differences, if any, between many of the treatment approaches discussed below (particularly presurgical orthopedic therapy). That research is important because, although two treatment approaches may provide the same long-term result, the burden of care (that is, the time and expense) associated with each one may be totally different.

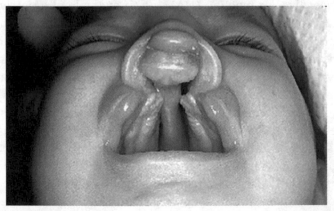

Fig. 5-5. *Dental arch collapse in an infant with bilateral cleft lip and palate. Reprinted (with permission from Elsevier) from Peterson-Falzone, S. J., Hardin-Jones, M. A., & Karnell, M. P. (2010).* Cleft Palate Speech. *St. Louis: Mosby.*

Presurgical Orthopedic Therapy

For children with complete cleft lip and palate, presurgical orthopedic techniques are sometimes used to mold (and/or retain) the tissues of the palate, gum ridge, and nose into their correct anatomical position prior to surgery. A variety of techniques may be used to bring the palatal segments into correct alignment.

A simplistic approach involves placing surgical tape across the child's upper lip. Taping can exert a force that will effectively move the underlying palatal segments back into a more normal position prior to surgery. When recommended, taping is usually carried out until just before lip surgery. Parents are instructed on how to tape the lip and may have to replace the tape throughout the day when it gets wet.

More elaborate presurgical orthopedic appliances, including active and passive appliances, are also used in some centers across the United States. Active appliances are dental appliances that move the palatal segments mechanically. They can either be removable or fixed (that is, surgically attached to the palate). They usually consist of two acrylic plates with an adjustment screw that allows the plates to be moved with controlled force. Passive appliances are retainer-like appliances that are placed in the child's mouth to maintain the distance between the two palatal segments while an external force (such as taping) is applied to the lip to move the alveolar/palatal segment into its proper place. Regardless of the type of procedures involved, any presurgical orthopedic approach taken requires frequent, careful monitoring to ensure that the right amount of movement occurs.

Nasoalveolar molding (NAM) is an example of a passive presurgical orthopedic procedure that is being used at some (but not all) treatment centers in the United States. Babies wear a retainer-like appliance to reshape the gum ridge and nose prior to surgery to minimize the severity of the cleft. (See Figure 5-6.) The appliance is created by an orthodontist soon after the baby is born and is continually modified (frequently on a weekly basis) in the months prior to lip surgery. Advocates of the procedure argue that children who receive NAM require fewer surgeries and have a better postsurgical result. Opponents of the procedure argue that NAM increases the burden of care (since numerous trips to the orthodontist are required and additional cost is incurred) and do not provide a better long-term result.

Although the use of presurgical orthopedics is one of the most controversial issues in cleft palate management today, reports suggest

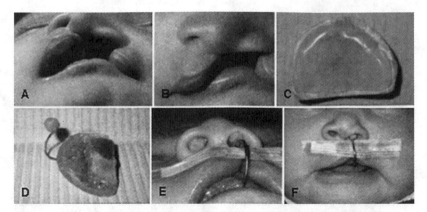

Fig. 5-6. *Presurgical nasoalveolar molding. A) Worm's eye view and B) en face view before treatment. C) Intraoral molding plate. D) Molding plate with nasal stent. E) Worm's eye view and (F) en face view of molding plate and stent in place. Reprinted with permission from: Ezzat, C. F., Chavarria, C., Teichgraber, J. F., Chen, J. W., Stratmann, R. G., Gateno, J., & Xia, J. J. (2007). Presurgical alveolar molding therapy for the treatment of unilateral cleft lip and palate: A preliminary study.* Cleft Palate-Craniofacial Journal, *44, 8–12, Allen Press Publishing Service.*

that the majority of cleft palate centers in the United States use some type of presurgical molding (Tan, Greene, and Mulliken, 2012). The surgeon and orthodontist on your child's cleft palate team can provide you with more information about this procedure if it is recommended for your child.

∷ Infant Feeding Plates

Some centers that use passive molding appliances claim that these appliances can minimize feeding problems and enhance early speech sound development in babies with unrepaired CP. Research has not supported these claims, however. Researchers in the Netherlands examined the use of these appliances and reported no differences in length of feeding, amount consumed, or growth between a group of babies who wore them during their first year and a group that did not (Prahl, Kuijpers-Jagtman, Van't Hof, and Prahl-Andersen, 2005). Similarly, our research has suggested that these appliances do not appear to facilitate consonant development in babies with cleft palate (Hardin-Jones, Chapman, Wright, et al., 2002).

Orthodontic Management

Children with repaired CLP have the same dental care needs as all children, but they may also have some special cleft-related problems that need treatment. For example, an orthodontist may be involved in your child's treatment early on if external lip taping and presurgical orthopedic appliances are used (as described above).

Later, orthodontic treatment will begin in the mixed dentition stage* when your child is roughly seven to nine years of age. Initially, the hard palate will be expanded (when necessary) using a palatal expander to bring the dental arches (and thus the teeth that are housed in them) into proper alignment. A palatal expander is a dental device that is used to widen the upper jaw to align the upper and lower teeth. Alveolar bone grafting can then be performed, if necessary, to repair the alveolar cleft. Orthodontic alignment of individual teeth using braces usually begins when most of the permanent teeth have erupted in the mid to late teens. This usually occurs earlier in girls than in boys. Correction of dental occlusion (bite) occurs at this time as well.

Palatal Obturators and Nonsurgical Treatment of VPI

Palatal obturators (plastic palatal plates) can be used to cover palatal fistulas and may be used to cover the hard palate prior to surgery for children who receive a two-stage repair. They can also be used as an alternative treatment for unrepaired palatal clefts when surgery cannot be performed due to concerns about the child's health (for example, if anesthesia is too risky due to a heart problem). They may also be used when the surgeon feels that surgery will not be successful (for example, if the palatal cleft is extremely wide).

When palatal obturators are used as an alternative

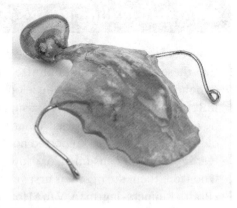

Fig. 5-7

---

* The mixed dentition stage is the stage of dental development when primary and permanent teeth occur together in the mouth—usually between five and thirteen years of age.

to palatal surgery, their design typically includes a palatal plate that covers the hard palate. Later, a tail-piece with an acrylic "speech" bulb on the end can be added to assist with velopharyngeal closure. (See Figure 5-7.) When used in children, these appliances must be modified over time as the child's mouth changes with growth. Routine visits to the dentist will be needed even in adulthood to make sure that good oral hygiene is being followed and to ensure the appliance is not compromising the health of the teeth or tissues in the mouth.

▪▪ Summary

The type and number of surgical and dental treatments that your child receives will be influenced by many factors, including the type of cleft he was born with as well as the philosophy of treatment held by the healthcare professionals on his cleft palate team. Whereas a child born with an isolated CL may need one surgery to repair the cleft (and perhaps one additional surgical procedure to improve the appearance of the lip and nose), a child with CLP will need three or more operations to repair the lip, palate, and gum ridge. When VPI is present, an additional operation may be needed.

An important benefit to having your child followed by a cleft palate team is that the professionals on the team can work together to develop a coordinated treatment plan for your child that minimizes interventions and optimizes outcomes. That plan will probably be modified over time, depending on how your child grows and the success or failure of specific interventions. In any case, you should have a copy of the expected treatment plan from your child's birth to tooth-jaw maturity, with updates as needed.

6

COMMUNICATION:

WHAT TO EXPECT DURING YOUR CHILD'S FIRST THREE YEARS

It is natural that you as parents of a baby born with a cleft palate (CP) might worry about how the cleft will affect speech and language development. You should know up front that some babies with CP have no difficulties at all after the palate is repaired. Other children have some delays in speech development, language development, or both that are treated with therapy or sometimes with additional surgery. However, rest assured that most children with CP eventually have speech that is perfectly understandable and in many cases indistinguishable from the speech of other children of their same age.

The ability to communicate using spoken language is one of the most important achievements of a young child's first few years of life. The process of language learning begins at birth, and by age three, children can typically carry on a conversation, produce a variety of sentence types, and make themselves easily understood, even though they may not produce all sounds correctly.

Parents play an important role in the speech and language learning process and can do a lot to help their children along the way. One of our motivations for writing this book was to tell you about specific things that you can do to help your child during these early years of speech and language learning (see Chapter 7). Our purpose in writing this chapter is to describe the communication accomplishments of these first three years of life and explain how these skills may be affected when a child is born with a cleft of the palate. We think that you will be interested in learning what to expect regarding your child's development and how to recognize signs of difficulties. That way, you can contact a speech-language pathologist (SLP) so that any delays in speech or language development are addressed as early as possible.

The information in this chapter about the development of language and speech in young children with and without cleft palate is based on research that has been conducted over many years. It is important to remember that these studies describe what is average or typical performance and to keep in mind that within every study population, some children do better and some do not do as well as this "average" child.

■■ The Beginnings of Communication

Babies learn language through interactions with their parents. And, long before babies can say their first words, they are communicating with lots of help from their mother and father.

Crying is one of the first ways in which babies "signal" that they need something. We do not really know whether parents can distinguish between cries of hunger, pain, and distress during the first few weeks of their baby's life. What is known, however, is that parents and other adults respond to babies' early cries and other vocalizations as if they are communicating. For example, when your baby wakes up crying, you might respond by saying, "Are you hungry? Let's get you something to eat." When you respond that way, you are acting as though your baby's "vocalization" (in this case, a cry) has purpose—that your baby is trying to convey that she is hungry. When parents do this, we believe that they are assisting the baby in developing *intentional communication* or in producing behaviors with the intent of communicating.

We do not know of any studies that have examined whether parents of children with CP respond in the same way to their babies' early cries and vocalizations, but we have no reason to believe that they do not. We have done some work looking at how mothers of children between twelve months and three years of age talk to their young children with cleft palate and have found that their interactions are very similar to those of mothers of youngsters without cleft palate. This is important, because from the start, parents need to interact with their babies with cleft palate just as they would interact with any other baby—that is, acting as though their children are communicating even though they might not yet be doing so intentionally

Intentional communication develops over the first year as the baby realizes that by communicating (e.g., pointing to or naming a desired object), her parents or other people in her environment can help her get things she wants or needs. Initially, a baby will communicate by crying, looking, or pointing to objects, but by about twelve months of age, she will begin to use words to refer to actions and objects she sees around her.

Two other important tools in the baby's communication repertoire are also developing during this early period. The first is *joint attention,* and the second is use of *gestures*. Joint attention, first seen when a baby is around ten months of age, is the ability to engage with another person around an object or event—that is, to deliberately pay attention to the same thing that somebody else is engaged with.

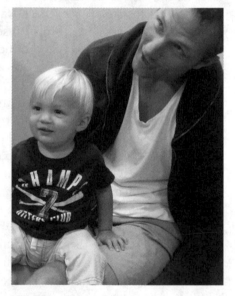

A baby's first attempts at joint attention are nonverbal. For example, a mother and her baby are playing with a baby doll. The mom gives the doll a drink from a cup and says (while looking at the doll), "The baby's drinking milk." The baby then follows her mother's gaze and looks at the baby doll. Eventually, gestures and then words are added to these shared interactions. For instance, the baby follows her mother's gaze, looks at the doll and the cup, and says "baby."

There is very strong evidence that joint attention helps babies to learn language, since we know that babies who are better at establishing joint attention are better at learning words.

Similar to joint attention, gestures are important to later language learning and provide a window on what babies are interested in. One of the most common early gestures is pointing, but babies also use gestures such as giving (giving a toy to someone else), pushing away (pushing away a spoonful of food), holding hands up (wanting to be picked up), or panting (to stand for the word "dog").

Studies of gestural development in babies and young toddlers suggest that early gesture usage is a good predictor of later language development. Babies who use more gestures early on have more words later on, and by watching the things that babies point to, we can predict the things they will eventually talk about.

We have no reason to believe that babies with CP have problems establishing joint attention, but there have not been any studies of this topic that we know of. However, Dr. Nancy Scherer, one of the authors of this book, has done research with several colleagues showing that toddlers with cleft palate who produce fewer words use more communicative gestures. This is good because it shows that even though toddlers with CP may not be able to say the words that they want to communicate, they are trying to communicate using gestures. When your child uses a gesture to call your attention to an activity or an event (pointing and looking at you when she sees a puppy playing outside) or to request (holding up her hands to indicate she wants to be picked up) it is important that you provide language to describe the event. In the first case, you might say, "Look, there's a puppy" while also looking from your child to the puppy, and in the second, "Oh, you want up" while picking her up. Eventually, as her language skills develop, words will replace gestures in these communicative exchanges.

Turn-taking is another communication skill that most babies develop in the first year of life. The earliest examples of turn-taking between a baby and parent are seen during feeding sessions. The "turns" occur when the baby stops sucking, the parent moves the nipple in the baby's mouth—then stops, and the baby starts to suck again. Turn-taking is incorporated into other games when parents pause after their turn, giving the baby an opportunity to take her turn. The baby's "turn" may include actions such as looking at the parent, kicking, and, finally, vocalizing. The early turn-taking sequences between baby and parent form the bases for later conversational skill development. See the box on the next page for additional examples of turn-taking activities.

▪▪ Examples of Early Turn-taking Actions

- Mommy tickles the baby's tummy, and the baby takes a "turn" by laughing. Mommy exclaims, "Oh, you want me to tickle you again" and begins tickling the baby again.
- Daddy plays "This Little Piggy" for a few seconds and then stops. After the baby wiggles her toes (considered to be a turn), Daddy begins again while saying, "Oh, you want to play piggies again."
- Mommy holds a blanket over her face, and when the baby pulls it down (considered to be a turn) says, "Oh, you want to play Peek-a-boo—Peek-a-boo!"

▪▪ Factors Influencing Early Communication Development

Professionals who are interested in understanding how babies learn language have identified some things that parents do naturally that help babies develop language more quickly during the first years of life. One area that has received a lot of attention is how adults talk to babies and how this "baby talk" differs from "adult talk" or even talk addressed to older children. This special way of speaking to babies is called "motherese," "parentese," or "infant-directed speech" (IDS). It includes using simple sentences, slowing down the rate of speech, and using exaggerated intonation patterns, facial expressions, or gestures. Additionally, when we talk to babies, we usually talk about the things that are happening or about to happen around us.

Interestingly, researchers have found that babies prefer IDS over the typical speech that is directed to adults, and that this preference is seen even if the language they are hearing is different from the language they are learning (e.g., French is the language being spoken, but the baby is learning English). Parents and other adults do not drop this special way of talking to children after infancy, but continue to use what is often referred to as child-directed speech (CDC) for just that reason. As you might expect, the nature of IDS changes as the baby gets older and acquires more language but is still characterized by exaggerated intonation and more restricted content.

Of course, there is lots of speculation as to why we use IDS when we talk to babies and young children. Based on many research studies conducted over many years, we now believe that adjustments that parents make in their language to babies and young children help them to learn the sounds, words, and grammar of their language.

Using infant-directed speech is not the only thing that parents do that may make language learning easier for babies. Researchers have identified other behaviors and techniques that parents use during natural interactions with their babies that are thought to promote language learning. These are described in the box below.

There are two important points to consider about these behaviors and their collective influence on language learning. First, most parents do these things naturally without any coaching. Second, if

▪▪ Parental Behaviors Thought to Facilitate Language Learning

Talking a lot	Talking often about things that are happening or about to happen (e.g., saying, "Let's take a bath now" while putting the baby into the bathtub).
Being responsive	Responding to a baby's vocalizations as though he or she is communicating (e.g., the baby babbles "dada." Mom responds, "Oh, you want Daddy?" and then calls for Daddy and says, "There's Daddy" when he appears).
Following the baby's lead	Labeling objects or events that a baby is looking at or pointing to (e.g., if a baby is looking at a rubber duck in the bathtub, saying, "Oh, you like that baby duck?")
Imitating	Responding to a baby's vocalizations by repeating what she said (e.g., responding to the baby's production of "duck" by repeating "duck").
Expanding	Expanding the content of a baby's production (e.g., Baby says "ball" while playing with the ball. Parent says, "That is a big ball").
Using IDS	Using a slow rate of speech with a slightly exaggerated, high-pitched, singsong quality. Using simple (but complete) sentences and simple vocabulary.

a baby seems to be developing language at a slower pace than other babies of the same age, it is not typically due to the way the parent(s) is or is not talking or responding to their baby. Still, a number of programs that employ these techniques have been developed for infants and toddlers who are having difficulty learning language. If you think your youngster is delayed in any of the areas described above, contact the SLP on the cleft palate team or an early intervention specialist in your area. Please see Chapter 7 for additional information on referral and early intervention services.

■■ Early Vocal Development and Babbling

During the first year of life, significant changes occur in the baby's sound development. At birth, a baby produces only *reflexive* vocalizations—such as crying, coughing, burping, etc. As the baby's lips, tongue, and other structures in and around the mouth grow and change, she begins to produce recognizable speech sounds.

Researchers have identified important milestones in sound development over the first year of life (see the box below). Some of the first vocalizations that babies make are *cooing* and laughing. Babies seem to make these vocalizations when they are "happy." Cooing consists of vowels such as "ah" and other vocalizations that sound as though they are coming from the back of the throat (such as the sounds "k" and "g").

The next stage that we see is called *vocal play* because the baby seems to be experimenting with different types of vocalizations (high- and low-pitched sounds, loud and whispered sounds, long vowel sounds, or raspberries made when the baby blows air through her lips).

Probably the most talked-about accomplishment of early speech development is *babbling*—the production of repeated syllables such as "bababa." Babies typically begin babbling when they are anywhere from six to nine months of age. Parents can easily recognize these babbled strings of sounds as speech. For babies born without a cleft palate, the sounds that are produced in these babbling strings are *m, n, b, d, g, w,* and *y.*

For most babies with CP, surgery to close the palatal cleft is performed around ten to twelve months of age. This is beyond the age range when we expect babies to begin to babble, and indeed, studies show that babies born with a CP may be a little slower to start babbling.

Also, sounds like *b* and *d* are difficult for babies with an unrepaired CP to produce since these sounds require holding air in the mouth and then releasing it to produce the sound (thus they are called *pressure consonants*). For a baby with a cleft, the air may escape through the nose instead of through the mouth. Rather than sounding like a *b,* the resulting sound will be closer to an *m.* It is important to remember, however, that babies with cleft palate can babble and that we can encourage babbling with sounds that are easier for them to make, such as *m, n, l, w,* and *y.* If a baby does produce a stop consonant such as *b,* it is fine to encourage that sound as well.

More specific information and activities describing how to stimulate babbling in your baby is provided in Chapter 7, beginning on page 108.

In some centers around the United States, babies are having their primary palatal surgery when they are around six months of age. It is not yet known whether these babies have more advanced babbling than babies who have their palate repaired later or whether their speech develops along a more typical timeline. However, studies are being carried out that will hopefully answer that question in the next few years.

Regardless of when your baby has her palate closed, it is important that you talk to her and treat her just like a baby without a CP by modeling and stimulating speech and language.

The final stage of sound development, *jargon,* refers to long strings of speech that sound like sentences but have no meaning. This stage overlaps with the next stage—production of words.

▪▪ Stages of Early Vocal Development

Reflexive Vocalizations	Birth
Cooing & Laughing	2–4 months
Vocal Play	4–6 months
Babbling	6–9 months
Jargon	10 months

☷ Early Comprehension Skills

While most babies may not say real words during the first year of life, they can understand many words spoken around them. By about ten months, babies can typically understand about forty different words. Some of the earliest words and phrases that a baby typically responds to are the following:

1. her own name,
2. "Mommy" (looks at Mommy when asked "Where is Mommy?),
3. "no," and
4. names for common objects such as "bottle."

Sometimes babies and toddlers appear to comprehend more than they do because they use context to help them understand. For example, after taking off your toddler's dirty clothes, you might say, "Let's put this dirty shirt in the hamper," and she responds by putting her shirt in the hamper. It is unlikely that she knew all the words in the sentence, but she may have understood a word or two and put the shirt in the hamper because that is the typical routine: taking off her clothes is typically followed by putting them in the hamper. If you had said, "Let's put the dirty shirt on the bed," she very well may have put the dirty shirt in the hamper since that is what you typically do with dirty clothes—showing that she does not really understand all the words in the sentence.

It is not just toddlers who use context to assist in understanding. We, as adults, do the same thing when we encounter an unfamiliar word; we use the words around it to determine the word's most likely meaning. Finally, most of us understand more words than we can produce. This is true for babies, young children, adolescents, and adults. Some common comprehension milestones over the first three years of life are provided in the box on the next page.

☷ Early Words

Sometime around twelve months of age (with the average range being ten to fifteen months) babies say their first real words. There is a lot of individual variation in the age at which babies produce their first words. However, if your baby cannot understand or use any words by eighteen months, you should consult a SLP.

▪▪ Comprehensive Milestones

8 months	Understands common phrase (e.g., "Give me a kiss.")
8–10 months	Understands common words (e.g., "ball")
10 months	Understands between 11 and 154 words
16 months	Understands between 92 and 321 words
18–24 months	Understands common two-word productions (e.g., "Kiss the truck.")
24 months	Understands yes/no questions (e.g., "Is this a doggie?")
30 months	Understands *what, where* questions (e.g., "What is she doing?")
30 months	Understands *in, on, under* (e.g., "Put the candy under the book.")
30+ months	Understands simple word order (e.g., "Mommy eats a cookie.")

Although there is some variability in the words that babies say first, the types of things they talk about with their first words are similar. First words are typically names of people or objects that they see and interact with every day. Common words that babies produce early on are *mommy, daddy, doggie, baby,* and *ball.* Most of a baby's early words are nouns, but she may also produce many non-noun words such as *no, more,* and *bye-bye.* While babies may know and be able to produce lots of words, some words are used over and over again and other words are used much less frequently. These words that are used frequently are also generally used in many different ways. For example, different uses of the word *ball* are described below.

A number of different factors determine which words a baby learns first. However, one important factor is the sounds, especially the first sound in the word. We know that babies are more likely to say words with sounds that are easy for them to produce and that were "practiced" in babbling. That is, they say more words beginning with *b,* such as *ball, baby,* or *bottle,* than words beginning with *s,* such as *sock, see,* or *soap.* Our studies show this is also true for babies with CP who have surgery

■■ Common Examples of a Baby's Use of the Word Ball

- Baby says "ball" as a ball is taken out of a bag.
- Baby says "ball" to request the ball that her brother is holding.
- Baby says "ball" while fussing and pushing the ball away to show that she does not want the ball.
- Baby says "ball" in response to Mommy's question "What's this?"

sometime around one year of age. Compared to babies without CP, who say more words with "pressure consonants" (e.g., *b, p, d, t, g*), babies with CP say more words with non-pressure consonants such as *m, n, j, l,* and vowels.

While babies seem to say words beginning with sounds that are easier for them to produce, their early words do not contain all the correct sounds and even all the right number of syllables. Their words resemble the adult words, but in most cases are not identical to the adult pronunciation. Because some words require more complex motor coordination than a one-year-old may be capable of, babies may do things like leave off a sound at the end of a word ("ha" for hot), leave off a syllable ("nana" for banana), or substitute a sound that is easier to say ("du" for shoe). If you have been around one-year-olds, you know that it is common to hear a baby say "dada" for daddy, "baba" for bottle, "ba" for ball, "dadi" for doggie, and "wawa" for water. A baby with CP who is attempting to say these words before her palate has been surgically repaired, may say "nana" for daddy, "mama" for bottle, "ma" for ball, "nani" for doggie, and "wawa" for water.

In addition to not containing all the correct sounds, a baby's early words may not be identical to the adults' in terms of their meanings. For example, sometimes babies use a word more broadly than an adult (they use the word *kitty* to refer to tigers, lions, and leopards) and sometimes more narrowly (they only use their word for blanket (*bankie*) to refer to their own blanket but not for the blanket on their parents' bed).

Most studies have shown that babies with CP are slower in learning to say early words. But they do not seem to have delays in comprehending new words. It is important to remember, though, that many babies with CP are not slower in producing words and may even be advanced in word learning. Although we do not know the exact reasons why some babies with CP are slower to add new words to their vocabulary, there are likely several factors including such things as otitis media and associated hearing loss and difficulty with sound production.

▪▪ Two Words and More

During the period of time from about twelve months to eighteen to twenty-four months, babies continue to add single words to their expressive vocabulary. They add somewhere between eight to eleven new words per month early on, and by the end of this period can say about fifty different words.

The point at which a toddler says about fifty words is important for two reasons. First, many toddlers experience a *word spurt*, during which they begin to learn words at a much faster rate. Some toddlers say up to twenty-two to thirty-seven new words a month. Second, they also begin to put words together to express more complex ideas. Some of these early word combinations consist of rote phrases such as "Inono" ("I don't know") that are really learned as a whole unit—not separate words. Others are actually two words used together to express a relationship between the words (e.g., "mommy hat" expressing the idea that the hat belongs to mommy). Some common *two-word productions* that occur in toddlers' speech in the second year of life are listed in the box below.

For some toddlers, the *two-word stage* is easy to identify, but for others it may be very short-lived and is followed very closely by the *mul-*

▪▪ Examples of Two-Word Productions

Possessor + possession	Hallie toy (e.g., Hallie's toy)
Person + action	mommy go
Action + object	throw ball
Person + object	baby bottle (e.g., baby [holding] bottle)
Person + location	Luke home
Object + location	ball floor
Object + attribute	ball big

tiword stage, in which the toddler produces strings of words such as "mommy go work" or "I see ball." (Hoff, 2009). Toddlers' early multi-word productions have been described by child language researchers as "telegraphic" because they contain the parts of speech important for meaning, such as nouns and verbs, but do not contain grammatical

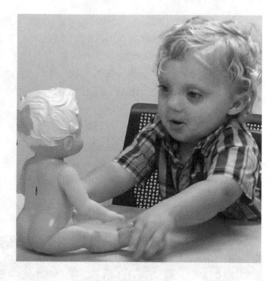

markers like -*ed* to express past tense or other words like *is* that may not be essential to understanding the message.

As toddlers learn more words and get better at stringing words together to form sentences, their speech production skills also improve. Although the process of learning all the sounds of the language continues into school age for many children, toddlers begin constructing the sound system of their language around two years of age. This means that although they are still not able to produce all sounds and words correctly because their motor skills may not be advanced enough, they are beginning to show consistencies in their productions of words with similar characteristics (e.g., the *s* sound in words is replaced with a *t*).

Many speech production patterns are commonly seen in toddlers during that second year of life and are therefore considered "normal." If they persist in older children, however, they are considered a problem. These patterns, along with the typical age at which they no longer occur, are listed below.

For young children with CP, speech development may be slower. This is because toddlers with CP may have begun producing words before their cleft was repaired or because VPI was present after surgery. Research shows that as a group, toddlers and young children with cleft palate may have the following difficulties with speech:

1. more difficulty being understood
2. more sound errors, especially on pressure sounds such as
   p, b, t, d, k, g, f, s

3. substituting sounds like *m* and *n* for other sounds
4. using the production patterns listed below for a longer period of time
5. producing sounds farther back in the mouth than is typical for sounds in English

The sounds that are consistently produced correctly by most preschoolers by age three are listed below:

Sounds Correctly Produced by Age 3
h, w, p, b, t, m, n, d, k, g, f*
*produced by girls but not boys

■■ Common Production Patterns and Age of Disappearance

Delete the final sound	"ba" for ball	Before 3 yrs
Repeat a syllable	"wawa" for water	Before 3 yrs
Delete a syllable	"nana" for banana	After 3 yrs
Sound becomes like another sound in the word	"kak" for take	After 3 yrs
If two sounds occur together, one is deleted	"poon" for spoon	After 3 yrs
Sounds produced at the front of the mouth replace those produced at the back of the mouth	"told" for cold	After 3 yrs
Substitute a sound that is easier to make	"do" for shoe	After 3 yrs

■■ Learning the Grammar of the Language

Around the same time that toddlers begin to put three words together (around age two to two and a half), they may begin to show the first signs of learning the grammar of the language. That is, in addition to using major parts of a sentence such as nouns, verbs, and adjectives, they also begin to use endings to mark tense (-*ed*) or function words (*a* or *in*) to complete the sentence. These parts of words or sentences are called **grammatical morphemes** and seem to be acquired by young children in a similar sequence. See the box below for a list of the grammatical morphemes that young children typically master by age three as well as morphemes that are developing (i.e., they are used but are not always used correctly).

In addition to learning these grammatical forms, young children begin to use sentences to ask questions ("What's your name?") and express longer sentences with more complex structures ("Go to the hospital and get it fixed like Papa John"—a two-year-old's response to her mother's comment "You're breaking my heart!").

▪▪ Grammatical Morphemes Mastered by Age 3

-ing	Baby cry<u>ing</u>
in	Baby <u>in</u> bathtub
on	Dog <u>on</u> bed
plural *s*	Two boy<u>s</u>

▪▪ Grammatical Morphemes Developing but Not Mastered until after Age 3

irregular past tense verbs	Baby <u>sat</u> down
possessive *s*	Mommy'<u>s</u> hat
is (as a main verb)	Baby <u>is</u> sick
articles *a, the*	<u>The</u> dog is running
regular past tense –*ed*	She wal<u>ked</u> home
regular third person *s*	He want<u>s</u> his car
irregular third person	He <u>has</u> my ball
is + verbing	Baby <u>is</u> cry<u>ing</u>
is contracted	Mommy'<u>s</u> sick
is + verbing contracted	She'<u>s</u> runn<u>ing</u>

Some preliminary evidence suggests that young children with CP are not slower to learn grammar or the forms listed in the box above, but they may produce shorter sentences. However, it is not clear whether they produce shorter sentences because of delays in language or because they think they will be more easily understood if they produce shorter sentences.

∷ Conversational Skills

While young children are learning the vocabulary, sounds, and grammatical forms of the language, they are also learning to be good conversationalists. We talked about the origins of turn-taking in infants in the section on the Beginnings of Communication above. As young children's language and cognitive skills develop, their ability to carry on a conversation typically grows too.

As we know, a good conversationalist responds to questions addressed to her and stays on, adds to, or begins a new topic appropriately. Additionally, a good conversational partner is able to adjust her language depending on her listener. For example, a preschooler with good conversational skills will use shorter sentences, a singsong quality, or rising intonation (IDS) when communicating with a baby or will speak more politely when talking to an unfamiliar adult than to another child.

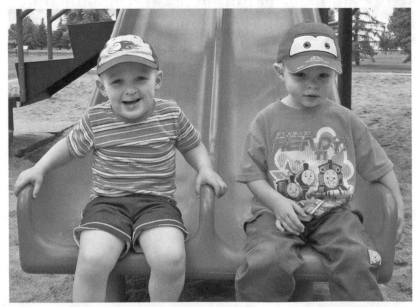

We do not know a lot about the conversational skills of young children with CP. But a few studies have suggested that three-year-olds with cleft palate may be less likely to initiate conversation compared to children of the same age without cleft palate. At the same time, they are very willing to respond to questions, even if they don't always add new information to the ongoing conversation.

When we studied the conversation skills of three-year-olds with CP, we found that children with more speech sound errors (and speech that was harder to understand) were less likely to initiate or add to the topic during conversations with their mothers or an unfamiliar person such as a SLP. It is our hope that toddlers and preschoolers with CP will be as willing as any child to engage in conversation with their family members, other children, and others they meet on a daily basis. Remediation of speech and language problems early on may help prevent situations in which young children do not initiate conversations because they are frustrated by their poor speech intelligibility.

■■ Baby Sign and the Teaching of Sign Language as an Intervention Technique

In the United States and other English-speaking countries, there has been a recent surge in the use of "baby signs" with infants who have normal hearing. This is an interesting phenomenon because for many years there was considerable debate about teaching sign language to hearing impaired and deaf infants. The thinking was that hearing impaired and deaf children needed to be able to get along in a hearing world and that using signs might make them less likely to learn to communicate using speech.

Today, baby signs are used with typically developing hearing babies to facilitate communication before they are able to produce spoken words. Proponents claim that baby signing results in more advanced language skills and higher IQs, better parent-child attachment and communication, and reduced frustration for babies. The benefits of baby signing have been reported in the popular media, and parents who use baby signs have been strong advocates, encouraging other parents to "jump on board." While it is not clear exactly how many parents are using signs with their babies, we do know that these signs have a short lifespan, and typically their usage decreases and then disappears as a baby begins talking. Numerous books, videos, and other materials are available commercially to show parents how to incorporate signing into interactions with their babies.

So, are the anecdotal claims about the benefits of baby signing true? Researchers have attempted to study whether or not baby signs or signing in general facilitates language and other related skills. Unfortunately, it has not been easy to prove the claims of proponents of baby signing. For example, not all studies of hearing babies of deaf parents have shown that the babies exposed to sign language at birth (along with speech) have better language skills than those exposed to speech only. Studies of the use of signs with hearing babies of hearing parents have not been well designed. Also, many of the studies showing positive effects of baby signing were actually carried out by the developers of the baby signing programs. A group of researchers from Canada published a review of all studies examining the effects of baby signing on toddlers' language development. These researchers concluded that there was no evidence that babies who were taught signs had advanced language development (Johnston, Durieux-Smith, & Bloom, 2005).

Signing may also be used by your baby's SLP as part of a vocabulary training program if your toddler is enrolled in early intervention. Not all SLPs think signing is a necessary part of intervention, and some even suggest that it should not be done. Instead, they recommend that speech-language intervention focus on actual speech and language production.

Researchers have tried to determine whether signing is beneficial for youngsters who are falling behind in speech and language skills. For example, studies have been conducted with toddlers and preschoolers with other types of communication impairments (e.g., children with Down syndrome). These studies have shown that using signs in conjunction with speech ("total communication") increases the child's communicative signs and spoken language and does not seem to decrease spoken language. However, the communication issues of toddlers with Down syndrome are different from those of toddlers with CP. Still, some SLPs may use signs as a bridge to speech for young children with CP who have language delays associated with the presence of a syndrome.

Before leaving this issue, we would like to emphasize one point. We cannot say whether teaching signs to hearing babies of hearing parents will increase, decrease, or have no effect on a baby's rate of language development. But, as noted by one group of researchers (Johnston et al., 2005), if you only have limited time and resources to give to your baby, perhaps your time may be better spent on things that we know will help with the development of speech and language skills. These strategies are discussed in Chapter 7.

▪▪ Bilingualism

Around the world, bilingualism is very common. In fact, approximately one-half of the world's population speaks more than one language. As a result, many children grow up being exposed to more than one language. While this is a less common occurrence in the United States, it is becoming more common. Recent statistics suggest that 21 percent of school-age children do not speak English at home (National Center for Education Statistics, 2009).

According to some experts on the topic of bilingualism, under the right conditions, learning two languages should not be difficult for a baby. Two things that are considered important to successful language learning, either of a first language or a second language, are 1) intact cognitive and language processing mechanisms and 2) a stimulating, language-rich environment (Iglesias & Rojas, 2012). That being said, it *is* more complicated to learn two languages at once rather than one. When a baby is exposed to only one language during the early language-learning period, the rules or patterns of the language she hears spoken around her are the same, regardless of who is talking to her. But if a baby is exposed to two different languages, some of the rules and patterns of the two languages may be the same, but others are different. The baby has to figure out which rules or patterns go with each of the two languages.

Interestingly, babies have the ability to distinguish between languages from birth, according to studies of infants who were exposed to two languages during the first year of life. Further, researchers are not convinced that babies who are exposed to two languages have delays in speech production or speech perception* that are due to bilingualism. Still, young children who are exposed to more than one language might be, but are not necessarily, slower in learning one or both languages (Conboy, 2012). For example, it has been shown that preschoolers who

---

* *The ability to identify and attach meaning to sounds.*

are learning Spanish and English simultaneously have more speech production errors compared to children who are learning English only (Gildersleeve-Newman, Kester, Davis, & Pena, 2008).

Over the last several decades, we have learned more about the language development of infants and toddlers who are learning two languages. As a result, some views about the wisdom of exposing a child to two languages have changed, especially if the child is at risk for speech and language delay. For example, it was once thought that if you wanted your baby to learn two languages, each language should be spoken by a different parent (or other person) in order to help her keep them separate. However, a number of studies have shown that babies can perceive differences in languages at an early age, so this strategy is no longer considered necessary.

Another recommendation that has recently come into question is advising parents of young bilingual children with communication impairments to only speak one language to the child and to conduct therapy in the "community" or school language, which is often the young child's second language. Speech-language pathologists sometimes suggest these measures, thinking that the child will have a better chance of improving her language skills if only one language is emphasized. More recently, however, recognized experts in the area of bilingual language learning have argued against this approach for a number of reasons. First, there is no proof that bilingual children with communication problems who are exposed to two languages have a more difficult time than children exposed to only one language. Second, continued use and growth of the home language helps to maintain cultural and family ties, which are important for a young child's social-emotional development. Yet, children also need to learn the language of the larger linguistic community. Thus, most experts now believe that if a child needs to be enrolled in intervention for speech and language problems, therapy should focus on improving speech and language skills in both languages (Kohnert & Derr, 2012).

To date, only one study has looked at language skills of children with CP who are learning two languages. The preschoolers in this study were living in Singapore and learning at least two languages (Mandarin and English) in school. When vocabulary skills were tested in both English and Mandarin, the preschoolers with cleft palate scored as well as preschoolers of the same age without CP on both English and Mandarin vocabulary tests. These findings suggest that learning more than one language is not any more difficult for preschoolers with CP than for other preschoolers. While there is still more that we need to know, at this point, there does not seem to be any reason to deprive a young child of the potential lifelong benefits of bilingualism (Young, Purcell, Ballard, Rickard Liow, Da Silva Ramos, & Heard, 2012).

If you choose to expose your baby to two languages from birth, you should know that even though both languages may be considered her "native language," she will not use either language like a child who is a native speaker of only one of the languages. This is because bilingual speakers process language differently as a result of being exposed to more than one language (Conboy, 2012). Your child may also be somewhat slower to develop skills in one or both languages due to differences in exposure, characteristics of the particular language, or just because of the presence of the cleft.

■■ Early Literacy Skills

Children do not typically learn to read until they start formal schooling. But babies who are brought up in homes where there are a lot of reading and other literacy-related activities going on show signs of emergent literacy skills as young as one year of age. What are emergent literacy skills? They are behaviors related to reading and writing that young children develop prior to the time when they actually know how to read and write. The emergent literacy stage starts at birth and continues until approximately five years of age.

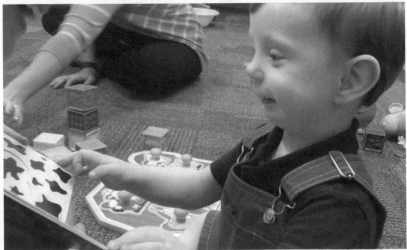

Some examples of *emergent literacy skills* include the following:

- knowledge about books such as how to orient a book for reading, how to turn the pages of a book, knowing that we read from left to right, etc.
- a young child "thinking" that she can read (pretend reading a familiar story), "reading" signs and other environmental print such as the sign for McDonald's, STOP (on the stop sign), or Coca-Cola (on the soda can)
- playing with crayons and other writing materials and acting as though this "writing" has meaning
- playing with or manipulating language as we do when playing rhyming games
- beginning to recognize the names for some letters

Over the past twenty-plus years, we have learned a lot about emergent literacy and how emergent literacy skills are related to later reading success. We also know that there are certain emergent literacy skills that "predict" later reading, writing, and spelling performance. They include the following:

1. alphabet knowledge or knowledge about the letters and the sounds they represent
2. print concepts or knowledge about how books and print are used and rules of print (e.g., how to turn pages, hold a book, read from left to right)
3. phonological awareness or knowledge of the sound structure of the language (e.g., knowing that words are made up of sounds, that *hat* and *house* begin with the same sound, and that certain words rhyme)
4. oral language skills (e.g., vocabulary, sentence structure or syntax, and story-telling abilities)
5. invented spelling or a preschooler's best guess of how something is spelled

Research has shown that preschoolers with strong skills in the areas listed above are likely to be good readers. In contrast, children with difficulties in these areas are likely to have reading problems. Notice that one of these areas is oral language skills. It might not be surprising to learn that children who have speech and language delays are at risk for delays in emergent/early literacy skills, reading, writing, and spelling. In fact, one study found that 53 percent of children with language delay during their preschool years had reading delays in second grade. In contrast, only 8 percent of children who did not experience preschool language delays had reading delays in second grade (Catts, Fey, Tomblin, & Zhang, 2002).

What do we know about early literacy and later reading in children with CP? Studies of older school-aged children with CP have suggested that, as a group, they have more reading problems compared to children of the same age without CP.

Only a few studies have looked at early literacy skills of youngsters with CP. One study that we carried out showed that the children with CP who had poor speech were at risk for delays in acquisition of early reading skills. In contrast, the children with CP and normal speech performed better on a test of early reading skills (Chapman, 2011). So, this is just one more reason why it is important to manage speech problems as early as possible, whether they are related to poor velopharyngeal function or not. Below, we have listed some skills that your child should have by three years of age.

:: By Three Years of Age, Your Child Should Be Able To:

1. say the name of several books
2. identify a few letters (capital)
3. look at books alone
4. scribble with a crayon on paper
5. recite a rhyme like "Pat a Cake"
6. realize that two words begin with the same sound

If your child is not able to do the things listed above by age three, talk with your child's SLP (if your child is enrolled in therapy) or the SLP on your local cleft-palate-craniofacial team. The good news is that there are many steps that you can take to facilitate these early literacy skills in your toddler. We have included activities in Chapter 7 that focus on this area of development as well as on helping your child acquire speech and language skills.

∷ Summary

This chapter provides an overview of the development of speech and language skills in young children from birth to age three and describes how specific skills may be affected by being born with a cleft of the palate. Of course, the precise effects will be different for individual children. However, we know that a CP always affects a baby's ability to make certain sounds (i.e., pressure consonants) in babbling prior to closure of the cleft. That, in turn, may affect her later speech and vocabulary development, as well as early literacy skills.

During this important period in your child's development, there is much you can do to assist your child as she acquires the skills described in this chapter. Chapter 7 describes some activities that you can use with your baby to enrich her communication and early literacy experiences, as well as considerations in finding and working with a speech-language pathologist.

Boosting Your Child's Speech & Language Development

Your child's speech and language development begins with you. The single most important thing you can do to encourage that development is...talk to your child...a lot. Although this advice may not seem very exciting, research has shown that the amount of talking that parents do with their children is important to later development. Toddlers from talkative homes tend to babble more than toddlers from less talkative families (Bardige, 2009). And the more a baby babbles, the more opportunities he has to practice and refine the consonants that will ultimately be used to form words.

In this chapter, we will talk about strategies to promote speech and language development that are effective when used by parents. We will also cover information about working with speech-language pathologists (SLPs), whether they are part of an early intervention or cleft palate team, in private practice, or at a university training clinic for SLPs.

Before we begin describing specific activities that you can use to stimulate your child's speech and language development, there is an important issue that we should address: the need to give your child a lot of practice in listening and responding to speech. Whereas older children will respond almost immediately to requests provided by adults, babies and toddlers need a lot of repetition before they begin responding in expected ways. Do not be discouraged if you engage your baby in an activity and the most he does is look at you. Just because he does not immediately imitate your actions or speech does not mean that he is not learning from the models you are providing. You will probably have to say a sound or word many, many times before your child attempts to imitate it.

▄▄ Early Intervention to Promote Speech and Language Development

The overall goal of early intervention (EI) is to identify, assess, and provide intervention as early as possible to lessen the impact of delayed development on a child and his or her family.

The United States Congress first mandated early intervention services for infants, toddlers, and their families almost thirty years ago. The federal government provides grants to the states to assist in setting up programs that will serve all eligible children and their families. Early intervention services are typically provided by a team of professionals from disciplines such as early childhood education, speech-language pathology, occupational therapy, physical therapy, special education, social work, nutrition, and nursing. The makeup of your child's team will depend on his profile of strengths and weaknesses.

If your child is experiencing a communication delay, he may be seen by either an SLP or a special educator or both. However, it is likely that the SLP will have input into developing the Individualized Family Service Plan (IFSP), which includes goals for your child as well as services for your family that will help you to support your child's development.

Early intervention services are typically provided in your home or your child's daycare (or the place where your child spends most of his time) on a weekly basis. The number of visits varies depending on the goals for your child and the level of family support needed. A major component of early intervention is collaborating with families, not only on planning the goals but in carrying them out. It is important that intervention or teaching not be confined only to times when a teacher or SLP is present, but that it be integrated into naturalistic activities.

(We discuss this in more detail below.) Therefore, parent training is a major component of the intervention.

All fifty states have early intervention programs. However, the eligibility requirements, the agencies that oversee EI services (the "lead agency"), and the cost to families varies from state to state. For example, in some states, any baby who is "at risk" for delays is eligible for services. In other states, the child must have 1) documented delays in one or more specified areas of development (e.g., feeding, communication and language, play skills, hearing, etc.) or 2) a medical condition that is often associated with delays (e.g., a syndrome such as 22q, Down syndrome, cleft palate, etc.). Also, the lead agency may be the Health Department, Department of Education, or Department of Rehabilitation Services, to name a few. Finally, while services such as assessment, development of the treatment plan (IFSP), and service coordination are available free to all families, you may have to pay for intervention services. For information about who to contact in your state, go to http://ectacenter. org/contact/ptccoord.asp.

Being born with a cleft lip (CL) or cleft palate (CP) will typically qualify a child for EI, but not all children with CP need early intervention services. As mentioned in Chapter 6, some skills such as production of pressure consonants will be difficult for a baby with an unrepaired cleft. However, if your baby understands everything he should for his age, vocalizes, and produces sounds such as *m, n, w, h,* etc., before his palate is repaired, EI may not be necessary. After palatal surgery, we expect a baby to begin to say sounds such as *p, b, t, d, k, g,* etc. (pressure

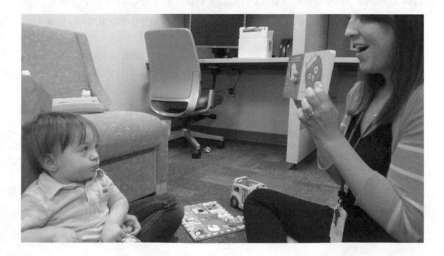

consonants). If your baby does not begin to say *b's* or *d's* (in babble or words) a few months after palatal surgery, you should contact the SLP on your baby's cleft palate team or an SLP working in early intervention. They will be able to tell you whether your child should be enrolled in an EI program. Either way, the activities described below are not meant to be a replacement for EI, but are appropriate for any child with CP, regardless of communication skills.

∷ Speech and Language Goals for Young Children with Cleft Palate

While no two infants and toddlers with CP have exactly the same strengths and weaknesses, our research and clinical work over the years have identified five goals or areas to focus on that are appropriate for a majority of children. Our goals for early intervention are different before and after palate repair. Prior to palate repair, we are more focused on promoting communicative interaction and vocalizations, but keeping in mind that some sounds may be difficult for babies with cleft palate to produce. Following surgery, our expectations change as we assume that normal speech development should be possible. Our goals then focus on stimulating production of pressure consonants (*p, b, t, d,* etc.,), expanding vocabulary, and eventually working on the grammatical forms that were described in Chapter 6, if speech and language delays persist.

The five areas we recommend focusing on are described below.

Increase the Amount Your Baby Vocalizes

Babies with CP, like all babies, need many opportunities to practice making different sounds and syllables. Practice is important because these practiced syllables turn into early words. For example, even before a baby uses "mama" to refer to his mother, he may practice "ma" or "mama" over and over again purely as sound play. In doing so, two things will occur. First, he will form a link between how the production sounds to him and how it feels in his mouth when it is produced. The more he practices this combination of sounds, the easier it is for him to "call it up" when he is ready to produce words. Second, he will begin to see the link between the production "mama" and what it symbolically stands for (his mother).

Babies who do not vocalize frequently have fewer opportunities to practice sound combinations and to receive feedback from their caregivers, both of which facilitate word learning. So, the goal here is to do whatever works to increase your child's vocalizations and to make vocalizing fun.

Increase the Number of Different Sounds Your Baby Produces

In our research, babies with CP as a group produced fewer (about one-half as many) different consonant sounds as babies without cleft palate who were the same age. A baby needs to produce a variety of different sounds so he can produce words that are readily understood by others. Additionally, babies who produce more different sounds when they are one year old are more likely to produce more words when they are three years old.

Increase the Number of Different Words That Your Baby Understands and Says

It is a well-accepted fact that babies with CP are typically slower at learning words, although the reasons remain unclear. (See Chapter 6.) Word learning is the basis for all later language development, so helping your baby learn more words will give him a better foundation for all language skills.

Increase Awareness of Air Flowing through the Mouth

When a baby has an unrepaired palatal cleft, his mouth and nose are not separated like they are after palatal surgery. Therefore, when a baby vocalizes or produces words before palatal surgery, air passes through his nose. Even after surgery, some toddlers continue to let air pass through the nose for all sounds. It may be necessary to help him understand that while the air comes out of the nose for some sounds such as *m* and *n,* the air should move through the mouth for most other sounds.

Facilitate Emergent Literacy Skills

As explained in Chapter 6, toddlers with CP (especially those with speech and language delays) may also be at risk for delays in early literacy and later reading skills. Most experts agree that it is easier to try to prevent reading problems than it is to intervene after a child has started to fall behind in reading (Rosin, 2006). So, the best approach seems to be to identify those toddlers who are at risk for reading delays and intervene early. Providing speech and language stimulation is one approach to facilitating emergent literacy skills. Also, many of the activities for increasing speech and language provided in this chapter can be modified to emphasize emergent literacy skills. We will provide guidance for how you might do that below.

▪▪ Stimulating Vocalizations

As mentioned above, we cannot expect a baby to repeat a sound or word after us. Instead, we have to *stimulate* or *encourage* him to make the sound. Initially, you are not going to be concerned with what your baby is "saying" but just that he is vocalizing. Researchers have observed infants and their caregivers and discovered that some routines are more likely to get babies to vocalize than others. For example, washing your baby's face or simply imitating his vocalizations may make your baby vocalize more. Here are some basic principles to think about when trying to encourage your baby to vocalize.

- *Observe your baby and determine the times of day when he is most vocal.* Take advantage of those times and plan your language stimulation activities accordingly. You may notice that your baby is more vocal in some positions than others. For example, researchers at Purdue University observed that three-month-old babies were typically more vocal when lying down, but that placing babies six months and older in highchairs did *not* encourage vocalizations (Nathani & Stark, 1996).

- *Make interactions face to face.* Depending on your baby's age, you want him to be lying down or sitting up, but he should always be facing you.

- *Use infant directed speech (IDS) when interacting with your baby.* Remember that this type of speech includes using exaggerated intonation patterns, a slower rate, and simple sentences. Infants prefer this type of speech, and it seems to help them with language learning.

- *Set up turn-taking routines.* Babies vocalize more and produce more advanced vocalizations when you respond to their sound attempts. Set up fun and motivating routines in which you take turns with your baby, and imitate all speech sounds that he makes during the routine to encourage more vocalizations. Show excitement every time your baby attempts to participate in the routine, and talk to him about what the two of you are doing throughout the activity. Start with something as simple as imitating each other as you stick out your tongues and make simple sounds. For older babies, the peek-a-boo game we have all played is a great turn-taking routine that progressively requires more participation from the baby. Initially, cover and then uncover your face with hands or a cloth without requiring your baby to do anything. After a few turns, leave your face covered until your baby vocalizes or actively uncovers it.

■ *Produce vocalizations such as raspberries and animal sounds.* These are "fun" vocalizations that your baby will enjoy making with you. Studies of babies interacting with their parents have shown that raspberries and other vocalizations may occur more frequently when washing your baby's face, and a baby may spontaneously make kissing sounds when playing with a baby doll. Babies also vocalize frequently when mouthing their hands, toys, or food. These situations may provide fun opportunities for you to elicit and imitate vocalizations from your baby (Rvachew & Brosseau-Lapre, 2012).

■ *Change it up.* Begin by imitating sounds your baby is already making and then add something new. If he produces a vowel-like utterance (e.g., *uh*), you could imitate *uh* and then add an easy consonant for him to say, such as "*m + uh*" or "*n + uh*." In Chapter 6, we described the sequence of vocal development, which begins with a baby producing basic vegetative sounds. See if you can identify where your baby is in this sequence and then try to take him to the next level. For example, if you hear your baby producing vowels, raspberries, squeals, or just sounds that seem to be "vocal play," imitate those productions and then try to stimulate productions from him at the next highest level. In this case, you might try to get him to imitate a syllable or strings of syllables such as "mamama" or "lalala."

■ *Incorporate the suggestions from Chapter 4 (page 53).* These are good techniques to use when interacting with your baby even if he does not have an ear infection or hearing loss.

■ *Do not reinforce glottal productions in your baby's early vocalizations.*
Babies, especially those with CP, may produce a cough-like sound
called a glottal stop (ʔ is the symbol that we use for this sound). A
glottal stop sounds like what you hear before the first vowel and
between the two vowels in the word "uh-oh" ("ʔuh ʔoh"). Babies
may produce long strings of vowels with glottal stops between each
vowel. They may also produce growls. If your baby makes either
glottal stops with vowel sounds or growling noises, do not imitate
those sounds, but model instead a sound that is produced within
the mouth (e.g., *m, n, l, w,* etc.). For example, if your baby produces
a glottal stop and vowel combination like "ʔa," you can respond
with "ma" or "wa." You could also ask, "What does a kitty say?" and
model "meow" without a glottal stop between the vowels.

❚❚ The Glottal Stop

In American English, we often produce a glottal stop as a
substitution for *t* in words of two or more syllables that end in *t*
+ vowel + *n* (such as bu<u>tt</u>on, moun<u>t</u>ain, and forgo<u>tt</u>en). When a
glottal stop is used in place of other consonants at the beginning
or end of words, however, it frequently interferes with our ability
to understand speech. Glottal stops produced by young children
with CP are believed to occur for two reasons. First, the child has
VPI and is stopping airflow to create sound in his throat before
air is lost through his nose, or he learned to do so in response to
previous VPI. Second, the child is having difficulty developing an
appropriate inventory of consonants.

❚❚ Stimulating Consonant Sounds

You can try to get your child to repeat any sound that you care to,
but be aware that some sounds and words may be more readily imitated
than others. Listen carefully to your child when he babbles and write
down all of the different sounds that you hear. As discussed in Chapter
6, the consonants that babies say during babbling are often those that
appear in their early words. That means that babies are more likely to
say a word when it begins with a sound they can already say.

Usually, as a child's spoken vocabulary gets larger, his inventory
of consonants expands as well. When possible, then, we usually prefer

to increase a toddler's spoken vocabulary in hopes that this growth will stimulate consonant growth as well. Sometimes, though, toddlers with CP attempt to say a large number of words using only a few consonants. For example, "ma" might mean "more," "mine," "mama," and "mouse." In such cases, a child's speech becomes increasingly difficult to understand as his vocabulary increases. When this happens, it becomes necessary to focus more directly on consonant production.

Although babies do not all choose to babble the same consonants, we can make several predictions about those that they will most likely imitate. Whereas babies without clefts most frequently babble *b* and *d*, many babies with CP do not produce these sounds until after palatal surgery. As discussed in earlier chapters, this is because these sounds and others like them that use a great deal of oral pressure require velopharyngeal closure. (See the list of high pressure consonants on page 157.)

Prior to palatal surgery (and even following surgery when VPI exists), when a baby produces high pressure consonants, air escapes through his nose. We believe that some babies with unrepaired cleft palate avoid saying these high pressure consonants because losing air through the nose results in loss of consonant identity. In other words, if enough air passes through the nose while saying *b*, it may sound like *m*. Similarly, excessive nasal air loss during production of *d* may cause it to sound like *n*. If your baby babbles either one of these pressure consonants (*b* or *d*) prior to palatal surgery, then you may want to try and stimulate the other. If you do not hear these consonants in your baby's babble, then you may want to begin by stimulating consonants that do not require high oral pressure such as *m, n, w, y,* and *l*.

In deciding which consonants to stimulate, you should also consider the structures your toddler is using for sounds he already says. For example, the consonants *m, w, p,* and *b* are made by bringing both lips together. If your toddler babbles "mamama" frequently, we might predict that he will more likely imitate another consonant that involves both lips—such as *w*. This does not mean that you should only stimulate the consonants that are easiest for your child to say, but use them as a starting place. Whenever possible, introduce new sounds in a meaningful way. If you want to work on *m,* for example, you can associate the sound with eating something yummy or babble the sound several times and then use it in a meaningful word such as *more* or *mama*.

Later in this chapter, we provide activities that you can use to help your toddler learn new sounds. Remember—you will probably have to say these sounds over and over many times before your child begins to imitate them.

▪▪ Readiness for First Words

Toddlers often signal their readiness to begin acquiring a vocabulary by imitating words. You may hear your child repeat words during play or conversation. But if you do not notice imitation, you can engage your child in an activity to set the stage for imitation.

As you read about the different techniques for helping toddlers produce sounds, words, and phrases, and even to acquire early literacy skills, you will notice that even though we might be talking about stimulating vocalizations in one section and building vocabulary words in another, many of the techniques are the same. For example, *turn-taking* activities are described in the section on increasing the amount of vocalization and *taking turns* in the section below on stimulation words. Other techniques, such as *expansion,* are also applicable to almost any interaction that you have with your toddler.

▪▪ Stimulating First Words

Several approaches have been developed to help toddlers learn words and sentences. Parents have successfully used two in particular to improve their children's language skills. The two approaches use similar techniques, and we will describe those techniques that have been shown to be most effective (based on research studies). Nancy Scherer (one of the authors of this book) and her colleagues have performed several studies using these techniques to improve speech and language of toddlers with cleft palate (Scherer and Kaiser, 2010).

The techniques we describe in this section are intended to be used in daily routines and play to promote communicative involvement. Toddlers are more likely to talk if they are involved in an activity. Once engaged, they are more attentive to language and speech input from others. These sorts of interactions provide excellent opportunities for toddlers to try to say new words. The strategies that are discussed below include suggestions for setting the stage for talking, deciding on what words to work on, and prompting techniques in routines and play.

Setting the Stage for Talking
Arrange the Environment to Encourage Communication

Children are more likely to talk when there is a reason for them to communicate. You can create that need to communicate through some simple organization of your home environment. That is, we recommend creating situations that require your child to talk about a problem or express a need. For example, here are some ideas for prompting communication related to toys:

- Put toys out of reach in clear containers or bags and rotate the toys in the containers to grab your child's interest. Choose some toys whose names begin with a sound that your child is learning. Wait for your child to point or vocalize before giving him what he wants. Repeat this activity or add new toys/items if you lose your child's interest. This sets the stage for using the prompting strategies that are discussed later in this chapter.

- Limit toys available for play. Put away some of the "old" toys as the "new" ones are introduced. Having too many toys/items out during these activities can reduce your child's attention to your speech. If he notices that the toys are gone, this is a perfect opportunity for him to request the toy!

You can also contrive situations involving food, clothing, or other household items that will inspire your child to try to communicate. The box/table below lists techniques you can use during interactions with your child to maintain his interest.

Play and Engage

Children learn best when they are interacting with another person. When you play with your child at his level, he is more likely to talk. Let him initiate the activity and lead the play. Avoid giving directions. Choose toys that are interesting to your child and put away toys that aren't being used.

You can make "play bags" by selecting several of your child's toys that go together in a theme and add a couple of other toys whose names

Technique	Example
Silly situations: do something unexpected	Use objects in unusual ways. Use a block as a hat, have a toy animal eat something inedible, make soup with unusual items.
Inadequate portion: provide small portions of desired materials	Give only a small amount of liquid in a cup or a small portion of a desired snack. Then wait for your child to request more.
Assistance: create situations where your child needs help	Put a shoe on your child's foot but don't tie it; give him a juice box he can't open.
Choice making: hold up two objects and see which the child wants	Do you want the ball or the car? A good way to introduce new vocabulary or words with specific sounds for practice.
Sabotage: not providing all the materials that your child needs in a desired activity	When setting the table, only give your child a plate and no cup or utensil; when playing with a toy basketball, put out the net with no ball.

have sounds you are trying to encourage. For example, put two cars, a small ramp, a ball, a truck, and a bike in a large zippered plastic bag. Place the bag where your child can see it, and wait a minute to see if he notices and requests the toys. If he wants to play, set up the ramp and start a race with the toys. This should give you plenty of opportunity to model words during play. Keep the toys in the bag when not playing with them to provide more opportunities for him to request more play time.

Notice and Respond

Notice and respond to all of your child's communicative attempts, whether he is using a gesture, a sound, or a word and whether you understand what he is communicating or not. Of course, if you understand what you child is saying, respond appropriately. For example, if he points to a ball out of reach, you can say "Oh, you want the ball? Here's the ball...ball," while giving him the ball. Providing your child with the object he wants is a natural reward for communicating. By describing your child's intent ("Oh, you want the ball"), you are letting him hear the words and the pronunciation of those words even if he was not able to say it all himself.

If you are not sure of his intent or if his words are unclear, make your best guess. Usually, if you are wrong, he will let you know! If you are having trouble understanding, you can ask him to repeat what he said. If that does not help, you might try to figure out what he is trying to communicate by having him show you what he wants; ask him—"Do you want the ball or the baby?" (while holding up each object in turn).

It is not uncommon for babies to use the wrong name for an object or to not pronounce the word correctly. In the first case, young children may "overextend" the meaning of words. For example, they might use a word like *truck* to refer to anything with wheels or *ball* to refer to all round objects. Because they don't have the words for all of these objects, they might really be trying to say, "That's like a ball." When your child does this, you can just provide the name and point out something that would help him to notice the difference between the two objects ("That's an apple. See, we eat it" while putting it up to your mouth and trying to eat). Depending on your child's ability level, you might then say, "Can you try that? Say apple?"

If your child mispronounces a word, you can also provide the correct model. For example, you can say, "Yes, **d**oggy," when your child points to a dog and says "goggy". Again, you have to use your own judgment about when you can ask your child to "try again" and improve the production. At the very least, you are providing a correct model of how the word *doggy* is produced. If you ask your child to modify his production ("Can *you* say **d**oggy?"), you want to be sure that you pick and choose when to ask him to do that. For example, if you know he can say a *d*, you might say, "Can you say **d**oggy?" while emphasizing the initial *d*. But, be sure that you do this sparingly. You don't want to break up the natural flow of every interaction by always asking him, "Can you say this?" or "Say that." If your child is being seen by a SLP, she will let you know what type of responses you can reasonably expect from your child.

Take Turns

Just as turn-taking routines can help increase vocalizations, they can also provide more opportunities to practice saying words. Your child will learn how to pronounce the sounds in words through practice. Like

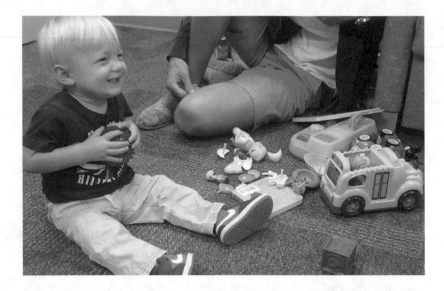

in a game of ball toss, conversation goes back and forth from child to adult and back again. So if your child starts the conversation, you respond and then wait for him to say or do something.

Balance the turns between you and your child. Respond to his actions, gestures, vocalizations, and words, but do not monopolize the conversation. Remember, sometimes children with cleft palate are less assertive in conversation. That is, they will respond to questions ("What's that?") or commands ("Say *doggy*"), but they may not be as likely to initiate conversations. If you are always asking questions or requesting a response from your child, he will not have the opportunity to initiate a topic of conversation on his own. Sometimes you need to be silent and let him take the lead in the conversation.

Practice balanced turns by saying one or two short sentences in response to each of your child's communication attempts. So, if he points to a car out of reach (which we consider taking a turn), you can ask, "Do you want the car?" Then wait for a response. If your child points again, you can model "car." Wait a few seconds to see if your child responds again. If he does not respond, you can get the car and another toy and ask, "Do you want the car or the ball?" When he responds with any vocalization or word attempt, you can model the name for the toy he chooses and reward him for his communicative attempts by giving him the toy. Again, if you think it is natural and appropriate, you can try to improve his pronunciation using the techniques described above.

Mirror and Map (M&M)

Imitate your child's actions with objects, and then "map" or describe what your child is doing. First mirror, then map. For example, if your child is pushing a car, you take another car and push it and say "Push the car." Mirroring and mapping is helpful when your child isn't talking. Of course you don't want to mirror behaviors that are unacceptable like throwing or hitting.

Imitate your child's actions with toys and wait to see if he notices. Provide a word or short sentence that describes the action. Change the activity and see if your child follows you. Map language onto the activity again and wait a few seconds to give him a chance to vocalize or use a word.

Deciding What Words to Work On

Choose words that begin with early developing sounds. A list of consonant sounds and words that are commonly produced by young toddlers is provided below.

Early Developing Consonant Sounds	Early Words
m	mama, me, mine
n	no, night-night
w	water, whoa
b	baby, boy, ball, bye-bye
p	puppy
d	daddy, doggy
h	hot, hi
y	you, yummy
t	tummy
k	cat (kitty), cookie
g	go, egg
f	fish, funny
s	sun
sh	sheep, shhh

Choose words that begin with sounds you have heard your child say. Remember, young children are more likely to say words that begin with sounds they have already practiced in babbling. Although the table above provides a list of sounds that usually develop early in speech development, the typical toddler will only produce a subset of these sounds. As previously mentioned, young children with CLP may have some difficulty using sounds that require high oral air pressure (i.e., pressure consonants) including *p, b, t, d, k, g, f, s, sh.* In addition, some children may make slower progress in acquiring speech sounds in general.

Your child's SLP can help you identify specific words to stimulate. If your child is not currently working with an SLP, then select one- or two-syllable words that begin with sounds that you have frequently heard your child babble. To begin with, it may be helpful for you to keep a brief diary of the different consonant sounds and words that your child says.

Prompting Words during Routines and Play

The more opportunities your child has to try to say a word, the more he can hear and compare his pronunciation to yours. Below are some techniques you can use to encourage your child to say words. Not all of these techniques work with all children. You will find that your child may respond to some when he is first starting to say words and others as his vocabulary increases.

| Modeling | There are two types of modeling: *Modeling 1:* Identify words that you want your child to say, and use them in your conversations with him. The more you use a word, the more likely he is to use it. So you can increase your child's vocabulary simply by using new words in your interactions with him. | If you want your child to say more words that start with *b,* use them while talking to your child, and he will try to say them. |

	Modeling 2: In addition to just using a word in conversation with your child, you can be more direct by asking him to say a word. This more directive form of modeling should not be used frequently, but it can increase the likelihood that your child will try a word when he is first learning it.	*Adult:* "Do you want to play ball? *Child:* (reaches for ball) *Adult:* "Ball." *Child:* (no response) *Adult:* "Say ball." *Adult:* "Do you want the ball or the truck?" *Child:* "Ball."
Expansions	Responding to your child by repeating what he says and adding a word or two is a good way to increase the complexity of his language. You can expand your child's gestures, vocalizations, or words and sentences. By adding words to your child's words, you can connect new words with words he already knows.	
	Gestures: Point/reach	*Child:* (points to ball) *Adult:* (points to ball) Says, "That's a ball. Ball."
	Give	*Child:* (gives adult car to drive) *Adult:* (takes the car) Says, "Give Mommy the car. Thank you."

	Vocalizations	*Child:* (makes bunny hop) Says "ah." *Adult:* (makes bunny hop) Says, "The bunny is hopping. Hop, hop, hop."
	Words	Child: (feeding a baby doll) Says "bottle." Adult: Says, "Baby wants a bottle. Bottle."
Speech Recasting	When your child is mispronouncing a word with his target sound, repeat the word emphasizing the target sound. Recasting provides helpful feedback to your child about his pronunciation. Encourage your child to try the word again, thus giving him another opportunity to say the word.	*Child:* Says "my" (for bye) *Adult:* "**B**ye-bye" *Child:* (waves) *Adult:* "Bye-bye"
Wait	To encourage your child to start the conversation, wait 1–2 seconds before starting the conversation. This gives him time to start the conversation. If he does not say anything, you can then model language for him.	*Adult:* (waits 2 seconds) *Child:* "Truck go."

▪▪ Play

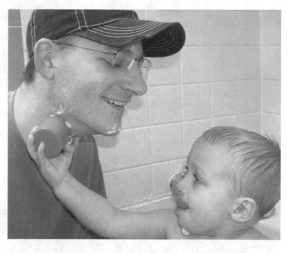

Why do we teach play? Linking words with engaging activities increases your child's opportunities to use words. Play is one of the primary activities that your toddler engages in. It can offer a foundation for prompting language.

Play often parallels language development milestones. Your child will use toys to replicate activities that he sees at home. His play may involve using toys in functional ways such as drinking from a cup or putting a comb to his hair. At this state of play development, your child will typically start to use single words. So we suggest that you model different actions and introduce new toys to your child's play. This should provide you the opportunity to "mirror and map."

As your child's play development continues, he will start to combine play into sequences that replicate routines he is familiar with, such as giving a doll a drink, wiping her mouth, reading her a book, and putting her to bed. This more advanced play stage often corresponds to the time when your child is beginning to combine words into short sentences. Your modeling and expansion can then emphasize short sentences.

When to Model New Play?

You should show your child new ways to play under the following circumstances:

- When your child keeps doing the same action with the same toy. For example, if your child likes playing only with cars, add some new toys like a truck and people or animals. Introduce these toys into the play. You can also change the activity by driving all the cars into a garage instead of racing them.
- When your child is doing an undesired action with a toy (e.g., eating Play-Doh or throwing toys). In this case, mod-

el a more acceptable use of a toy (give your child a bucket to throw toys into rather than throwing them in the air or at you). We use an indirect approach at first to redirect a child's play, but if he continues to use the toy inappropriately, we say, "No throwing the toys" and then change the activity entirely to give the child a positive option.

Expanding Your Child's Vocabulary

To help your child learn new vocabulary, you need to help him make the connection between the words and the objects or routines he is interested in. When your child is involved in an activity that holds his attention, describe what he is doing using simple sentences. For example, if he is feeding the family cat, you can comment on the activity by describing what is going on: "Kitty is eating" or "Luke is feeding the kitty." You can also use this as an opportunity to further expand your child's vocabulary of words that have speech sounds that he should be using. These words are called target words and often include words that have early developing sounds. (See the box on page 115 of this chapter). If your child is receiving early intervention services, his SLP can also help you choose these target words, continually expanding that list as your child develops.

Here is an example of an activity that can help your child learn new vocabulary and new sounds. Let's say that your child is working on target words that contain the *k* sound, such as in the word *kitty*. You can copy your child's play with a toy that has his target sound. If he is feeding a kitty, you can start feeding a cow. Then give your child the toy. If he plays with the toy, model the target word using short, simple sentences. For example, if your child tries to say "cow" when you are feeding the cow, you can repeat what he says (e.g., "I am feeding the cow. Cow") and keep the conversation going back and forth a few times before your child's interest changes.

:: Transitioning into Word Combinations

When children are able to use about fifty different words, they are typically ready to start combining words to form two-word phrases such as "Mommy hat" (i.e., *That is Mommy's hat*) or "Mommy run" (i.e., *Mommy is running*).

Dr. Chapman and her colleagues were interested in determining if they could help toddlers who were already producing lots of single words to combine those words into two-word phrases using naturalistic activities similar to what parents might do. They found that after a short period of training, more than 50 percent of the children increased their ability to put two words together. We will therefore describe their method here so you can help your child learn to make two-word phrases.

The method involved using a question-and-response type of interaction and expansions (see below) while looking at pictures or acting out events using toy dolls and objects. A picture book was designed (using pictures from coloring books or other sources appropriate for the child's age) and toy objects were selected to act out different two-word combinations based on the child's vocabulary (e.g., person + object = "baby juice" for *baby drinks juice*; object + location = "baby bed" for *baby is on the bed*; possessor + object = "Mommy hat" for *Mommy's hat*). In an attempt to make this training as close to typical language learning as possible, we used a questioning technique similar to what occurs naturally between a toddler and his parents. Below is an example of the exchange that might occur between you and your toddler.

:: Sample Conversation Showing How to Encourage Multiword Combinations

Adult: "Who's that?" (Pointing to a picture of a mother or mother doll for the enactment)

Toddler: "Mommy."

Adult: "Yes, that is Mommy."

Adult: "What is she drinking? (Pointing to a picture of juice or the toy juice for the enactment)

Toddler: "Juice."

Adult: "Yes" or "Right." "Mommy juice" or "The mommy is drinking juice." (While pointing to each of the pictures or objects)

When helping your child learn to put two words together, it is best if he already knows both words in the two-word combinations. This way he does not have to learn the meaning of the words but can focus on the relationship between the two words. You can also model and try to facilitate two-word combinations during activities like putting toys in the toy box as part of your normal day.

Mom: "Who is this?"
Response: "Baby."
Mom: "Yes, that is the baby."
Mom: "Where is the baby going?"
Response: "In."
Mom: "Yes, baby in. The baby is going *in* the box."

Repeat with each toy going into the toy box.

▪▪ Books and Music to Stimulate Language and Emergent Literacy Skills

Books

Reading aloud to your child and talking about pictures in books is a great way to expand his vocabulary, develop listening skills, encourage imitation, and facilitate emergent literacy skills. Your toddler will not understand all the words you say when reading aloud. But sharing books provides multiple opportunities for him to associate words with pictures, sounds with letters, and sequences of sounds with specific words.

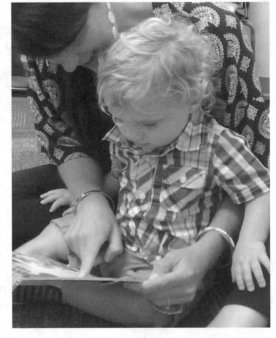

These shared reading activities also provide opportunities for your toddler to learn about print concepts (how we hold a book, what books are for, etc.). So, make reading part of your daily routine whenever possible. Keep a basket of books in each room that your child spends time in to encourage reading.

Many babies begin paying attention to pictures in books by age six months, and, by their first birthday, many babies begin to actively point to pictures and also follow simple directions (such as "Pat the bunny") and imitate animal sounds (Bardige, 2009).

When shopping for books, bear in mind that books with photographs of other babies and toddlers are particularly intriguing for young children. Look for ones that provide an opportunity for your child to:

- name common objects, people, and body parts,
- imitate actions (such as clapping and waving),
- imitate routines (peek-a-boo),
- learn the alphabet symbols and the sounds they stand for (ABC books),
- focus on rhyming and play with sounds.

Since toddlers are hard on books, make sure you purchase durable editions. Look for books that will be easy for your child to hold with colorful pictures of common objects and people that are involved in daily activities. Avoid books with lots of words.

Although we enjoy reading stories to our children, it is important to remember that "reading a book" with your child is an experience that will change over time as his knowledge of the world and ability to express ideas changes. Initially, he may only be interested in chewing or banging books. Even once he begins looking at books, he may be more interested in turning the pages than in actually looking at the pictures...or he may be more interested in the pictures than in the story that accompanies them.

Let your child guide the activity and enjoy the shared experience with you. Over time, you will be able to identify the books that he likes the most and will learn the routine that he prefers. It is not a problem if your toddler wants you to read the same book over and over. In fact, that will help him to learn the vocabulary, and then when he is a little older, it will be easier for him to understand the story and then be able to tell the story back to you. Whereas some children enjoy turning each page and looking briefly at the pictures, others may turn to specific pages of interest, and their strategy for "reading" may change with different books.

Interactive books that allow toddlers to do more than just look at pictures are particularly good choices. Many such books are on the market today and encourage toddlers to poke their fingers through holes, touch different textures, lift flaps, and look in mirrors. Homemade books that include photographs of family members and pets are often favorites as well.

You will notice that many of the recommended books listed below have repetitive words or phrases and stories that are very predictable. This is also important for development of emergent literacy skills, as toddlers are able to participate more easily in the shared reading activity and are excited if they can "fill in" the words or tell "what is going to happen next." Finally, many of these books have lots of words that either begin with the same sound or rhyme. Those books are great for developing phonological awareness skills in toddlers.

Finally, as with many things in life, timing is everything! If you are trying to identify a good time for reading in your routine, choose a time when your child is most likely to take the time to look at books. Reading just before naps, after baths, and bedtime is always a good

‖ What If My Child Is Not Interested in Books?

We know that about 10 percent of young children are not interested in reading books, and some even refuse to participate in book-sharing activities (Kaderavek & Justice, 2002). Reading experts suggest that you should not try to force toddlers to "read" books if they are not interested. However, there are things that you can do to make reading activities more interesting and fun for those toddlers.

If your child is always on the move and does not show an interest in books, then gradually make books a part of his routine by introducing them into specific play activities. For example, show your child a picture of a monkey in an animal book and then act like a monkey together. Prompt him to pick another animal in the book to imitate. You might also try having toys as props for the story to heighten interest. Having a puppet read the story or finding books about favorite activities or something your toddler really loves to do might motivate your toddler's interest in books (McWilliams, 2006).

time to capture your child's interest because his energy level is lower and he is less focused on *moving*. That said, we believe that any time your child brings a book to you to look at is a good opportunity for reading. And books provide a good foundation for early language and literacy development.

A few books that we have used with toddlers (including our own) that provide simple language (if any), lots of repetition, and/or interactive activities are listed in the table below (and can be found in most bookstores). This is not an exhaustive list, and there may be other favorites that you or your child prefers.

Print Concepts

Now we are going to talk about some strategies that you may incorporate into your shared reading activities that will facilitate emergent literacy skills, specifically print concepts. First, you want to sit close to your child or have your child on your lap. You want to be sure your child is engaged and paying attention! Second, there are lots of things that you can do to "teach" print concepts:

- Before you start reading, say the title of the book, and say who the author is. At the same time you are saying these things, you can also point to the title and author's name.
- You can talk about the front and back of the book as well as how the book opens and closes.
- When you are actually reading the book, you can point out the relationship between the pictures and words, especially in books that have the names of the pictures written out. For example, when you point to the picture of a baby, also point to the word *baby*, while saying, "This says baby."
- When your toddler is a little bit older, you can point out similarities between words with the same beginning sounds, so you might point to the *d* in *duck* and *doll* and say, "See, both words start with *d—duck* and *dolly*." Or, "That word starts with *h*—just like your name—Hallie."
- When you are reading books with more words, it is good to run your finger under the words as you read.
- Finally, when the story is over, say "THE END"!

■ A Few Recommended Book Titles

Title	Author	Comments
Baby! Baby!	Vicky Ceelen	No words; Pictures of babies and animals in similar poses
Belly Button Book	Sandra Boynton	Lots of *b* words
Blue Hat, Green Hat	Sandra Boynton	Good book to encourage two-word sentences. Focuses on a turkey. getting dressed. Introduces colors. The refrain "oops" is repeated throughout.
Brown Bear, Brown Bear	Eric Carle	Colorful pictures Repetitive phrase: "What do you see"
Click, Clack, Moo, Cows that Type	Doreen Cronin	Repetitive phrase: "Click, clack, moo"
Cock-a-Doodle-Moo	Bernard Most	Lots of repetition
First 100 Words boardbook	Priddybooks	Colorful pictures of common foods, clothes, toys, animals, and actions
Five Little Monkeys	Eileen Christlow	Repetitive phrase: "No more monkeys jumping on the bed"
From Head to Toe	Eric Carle	Encourages imitation of animal movements
Is Your Mama a Llama?	Deborah Guarino Steven Kellogg	Rhyming Repetitive phrase: "Is your mama a llama?"
MaMa MaMa	Jean Marzollo	Repeats phrase "MaMa, MaMa"

Moo Baa, lalala	Sandra Boynton	Good book to encourage single words. Focuses on sounds that animals make. Simple words that most babies can say.
Papa Papa	Jean Marzollo	Repetitive phrase: "Papa, Papa"
Tickle the Duck	Ethan Long	Different textures to touch
Where's Spot?	Eric Hill	Simple colorful pictures; "Lift-the-flap" book; Repetitive phrase: "No"

Prompting and Question Strategies

Experts in the area of emergent literacy have described prompting and questioning strategies that you can use with your child during a sharing books activity (modified from Lonigan & Whitehurst, 1998; McWilliams, 2006). See below.

Complete the sentence	This prompts the child to fill in a word. "Five little monkeys jumping on the ____." (bed)
Recall questions	Ask a question related to the story. "What happened to the monkey?"
Open-ended questions	Helps to increase talking during shared reading. "What's on his head?"
Wh questions	Expands vocabulary. "What do you think ____ means?"
"Distancing" questions	Helps your toddler relate actions in the book to his experiences. "Do you remember when you bumped your head? What happened?"

In addition to asking these types of questions, you will want to evaluate your child's response to the questions and provide feedback ("Right, he bumped his head!"). As with other language learning activities, you can expand what your child says ("Yes, he bumped his head when he fell off the bed!"). Finally, during the next reading of the book, you can ask the same question ("What happened to the monkey?"). While questioning is an important tool for increasing vocabulary and other aspects of language, you don't want to overdo the questioning. You want the questions to be a natural part of the interaction.

Model Literary Skills for Your Child

Young children learn a lot by observing what goes on around them, and they love to "play" at things that Mommy and Daddy do such

---

❖ Other Things to Incorporate into Your Book-Sharing Activities

Make reading fun for your toddler by using exaggerated intonation patterns and changing your voice (including pitch and loudness) for different characters in books. This will help to grab and keep your child's attention.

Use shared book reading to work on sounds or vocabulary words. You can emphasize words with sounds that your child is learning as you read together. For example, emphasize or stress the sound or word that you want your child to attend to. You may first want to have your child show he understands new vocabulary words by having him "Find the duck" in the picture. The next step would be to have him label the duck or respond to questions concerning the duck. The next time a duck appears in the story, you could point to it and say "What's that?" If your child provides the appropriate word, act excited and reinforce the name by saying "Yes, that's a duck." If he uses the wrong name (e.g., calling a duck a chicken), don't just say, "That's not a chicken." Your child is more likely to learn the name if you point out a difference between the two objects. In this case, you might say, "That's a duck. He says quack-quack."

When you think your child is old enough, you can begin to have him tell you the story, maybe just going back through the pages initially and asking him what occurred on each of the pages. As he gets older, you might try having him act the story out with props or have him tell you the story and write it out for him.

as pretend shaving, blow drying their hair, cleaning, or carrying out activities with a baby doll. For this reason, we want to model reading and writing activities for our young children.

Let your toddler see you read. Draw attention to words that you see frequently in your home (e.g., labels on foods), on the way to preschool or daycare (e.g., stop signs and street signs), or in your neighborhood (e.g., store logos).

When you write things, show your toddler and describe what you are doing. Let him "write" by providing lots of opportunities for drawing with pencil and paper, crayons, chalk and chalkboard, finger paints, shaving cream, etc. Write thank-you notes or letters, grocery lists, and menus, even if your child only makes a mark on the page. If your child draws a picture, label the picture for him, and see if he can tell you a story about it that you can write down.

Music

Have you ever noticed that most toddler shows on television are loaded with music? Whether the children are dancing or marching to music, they are usually singing a simple song that is repeated time and again on the show. Our children are now grown, but we still remember the shows they watched as toddlers largely because of the songs that we cannot get out of our heads! We remember, too, the first time we looked up and saw them imitating the movements of the kids on those shows.

Toddlers instinctively begin moving when they hear music. And movement encourages many quiet toddlers to babble or talk. Make time for music in your daily routine. Whether you are bouncing your child on your knee, chanting simple nursery rhymes, or singing along with a DVD, you are helping him develop rhythm and coordination while also providing an excellent context for language development (and emergent literacy skills) to occur.

■ Increasing Oral Airflow

Normal speech production requires air to pass into the nose for nasal consonants (such as *m* and *n*) and into the mouth for other consonants. Recall that prior to palatal surgery, a baby with CP has no separation between the mouth and nose. When a baby babbles or says a word, air passes into his mouth and out the nose. Some toddlers who have had their palate repaired do not understand that air can now go

▪▪ Apps Everywhere!

There are a number of apps on the market that have been developed for use with babies and young toddlers. As SLPs, we feel that a word of caution about their use is appropriate. Although we support the use of educational apps in early intervention, we do not consider them to be an adequate substitute for personal interactions or the play that is so important to a toddler's discovery of the world. We believe apps are one of many tools that can be used effectively with toddlers to promote good speech and language development if the following conditions are met: 1) they are developmentally appropriate, 2) they are used sparingly throughout the day, 3) they are used with adult supervision.

When selecting apps for your child, look for simple, interactive ones that contain large, colorful pictures. They are often more engaging than those that have more complex (busy) illustrations. As with books for this age group, select apps that have repetitive (and thus predictable) actions—preferably apps that include familiar routines (feeding baby, saying hi/bye-bye, eating), people (mommy, daddy), animals, and toys that your child encounters each day. *Talking Hippo* is a good example of an app that can be used to promote imitation in a young toddler.

through either the nose or the mouth to produce different sounds. They actively compress their lips together and snort air through the nose to produce some sounds.

Simple airflow activities (such as blowing party horns) can help a child: 1) feel the difference between nasal and oral airflow, and 2) learn to direct air through the mouth. Activities that can be used with young children to teach the concept of oral airflow are provided in the next section (see Blowing Party Horns and Bug Race). In each activity, children are asked to either blow a horn or produce an explosive sound with their lips. For a child's first attempt, we hold his nose so that all air is physically directed through the mouth. After several attempts, we may keep our fingers on the side of the child's nose but not pinch the nostrils together to see if he is purposefully directing air through the mouth.

When using these activities, it is important to remember that most toddlers with repaired cleft palate have the ability to achieve velopharyngeal closure. Thus, our goal with airflow activities is simply to show them what they are already capable of doing. If your child has VPI, it may be more difficult for him to achieve success. Since these activities are only designed to teach the concept of oral vs. nasal airflow, they should be discontinued if a child repeatedly fails to produce the desired result independently.

A Helpful Resource: Kristi Chamberlain, an SLP, has written the *Early Articulation Books for Cleft Palate Speech* series (www.linguasystems.com/). The series includes six spiral-bound books that focus on a chipmunk named Chippy. Chippy has difficulty producing oral airflow and saying the pressure consonants. Each book describes how his sister Twitch helps him learn to either direct airflow orally or produce specific consonant sounds (*h, f, v, p, b, t, d, k, g*). These are cute, simple books that you can read and talk about with your older toddler if he is having problems saying these sounds.

▪▪ Can Blowing Simple Party Horns Increase Muscle Strength?

Some speech-language pathologists believe that blowing simple party horns can help children strengthen the speech muscles. This is a highly controversial practice that is not supported by research. Not only is there a lack of evidence demonstrating that these activities can increase muscle strength, but children with isolated CP do not have muscle strength problems to begin with! So why do so many SLPs use horns? We suspect there are many reasons why they are popular. Some SLPs may believe that a cleft palate results in muscle strength problems. Others may engage a child in blowing activities because they can obtain a quicker response if they ask a child to blow a horn than if they engage him in speech-language-based activities designed to expand his vocabulary.

Regardless of their rationale, we believe that the use of blowing activities to increase muscle strength in therapy is a waste of time—time that is better spent working directly on speech and language. Since toddlers with isolated CP do *not* have problems related to muscle weakness, *party horns should only be used to help toddlers understand the concept of oral airflow.*

▪▪ Activities to Stimulate Vocalizations, Consonants, and Early Words

Encouraging Vocalizations 1

> **Purpose:** Encourage vocalizations
> **Items Needed:** None
> **Target Group:** Babies

Instructions:
- Place your baby sitting up on your knees, lying down on your knees, or lying on the floor. Be sure you have your baby's attention and tickle his tummy or wiggle his toes to elicit some type of vocal behavior such as laughing or cooing. While tickling, describe what you are doing ("Tickle your tummy") using simple language addressed to your child. Imitate your baby's vocalization. Then say, "You want me to tickle your tummy?" while you tickle his tummy again. Try to keep this game going for a few turns. Be engaging and make it fun for your baby. Show excitement and pleasure when he "takes his turn" by vocalizing.

Encouraging Vocalizations 2

> **Purpose:** Encourage vocalizations
> **Items Needed:** Clear jar with a lid; small toys that fit inside but are too big to swallow
> **Target Group:** Babies who are babbling or producing single words

Instructions:
- Put some attractive/desirable toys into a clear plastic jar, shake it, and then hand it to your baby.
- Wait for your baby to "ask" you to open the jar. Depending on your baby's level of language usage, you can expect different

behaviors to "request" that you open the jar. At the very least, you want some type of vocalization to accompany any gesture that your baby uses to indicate that he wants help.

▪ If your baby produces a gesture only, model a word such as "open" or "help" for him to imitate. Do not open the jar until he has produced some vocalization to indicate what he wants you to do. You can shake the toy, point to the toy, etc. to encourage a vocalization. After your baby vocalizes, model a correct word such as "open" and then expand "you want me to open the jar" as you open the jar. If your baby produces a word such as "open" or "help," imitate the word and then expand on it (e.g., "open"—"Oh, you want me to open the jar.")

Variations:
▪ Place Cheerios in a jar that your baby cannot open. Follow the procedures above. Let him eat some Cheerios after he vocalizes.
▪ Place a juice box (that your baby cannot open) and a cup in front of him. When he requests juice, place some in the cup, but don't fill it up. This way your child can have an opportunity to request more. Follow the procedures above.

Bouncing Baby

Purpose:	Encourage listening, vocal play and imitation
Items Needed:	None
Target Group:	Babies who are babbling or producing single words

Instructions:
▪ Bounce your baby on your knee. As you hold your baby, let him/her "fall" through your knees or "fall" to one side. Say "whoa!" As you pull your baby upright, say "up!"
▪ After repeating this activity several times, let your baby "fall" through your knees as before, but this time just look at your baby expectantly. Wait for him to vocalize or say "uh oh." Repeat what he says, and then repeat the activity.

Mirror Talk

Purpose: Encourage listening, babbling, and imitation
Items Needed: Mirror
Target Group: Babies who are babbling or producing single words

Instructions:
- With your baby on your lap, look in a mirror and make funny faces (examples: stick out your tongue, pucker lips, smack lips). Encourage your child to imitate the movements.
- Pair a sound with the faces/movements and encourage your child to imitate both. Examples: stick your tongue out and make a raspberry sound, pucker lips, say "oo, oo, oo," pretending to be a monkey.

Book Reading

Purpose: Motor imitation, vocal imitation, emergent literacy
Items Needed: Small photo album, pictures of your baby and family members
Target Group: Babies who are babbling or producing single words

Instructions:
- Create two small photo-album books for your baby. One book should include pictures of your baby doing routine activities such as eating, bathing, playing, having diaper changed, etc. The other book should include photos of family members and pets.
- With your baby on your lap, look at the pictures in each book and talk about/label them using simple language

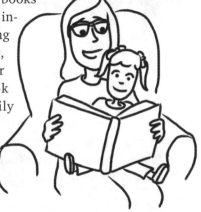

("Hallie's bottle," "Hallie is eating," "Hallie is playing," "Hallie is washing"; "Daddy goes bye-bye"; Hi, Mommy").
■ After you and your child have looked through the book several times, pause periodically after turning each page to see if your child will comment on the pictures.

Singing

Purpose: Encourage listening, babbling, and imitation
Items Needed: MP3 player, CD player, or musical instrument
Target Group: Babies who are babbling

Instructions:
■ Play a song that your child enjoys.
■ Sing "la" for each of the words in the song. Since many babies babble more frequently when they are moving, bounce to the music while you sing "lalala!"
■ If your baby attempts to sing along using a different syllable (such as "*mama*"), repeat that syllable as you sing to the tape.
■ After 10 or more repetitions of the syllable, change to another syllable (such as "dada") and see if your baby will imitate the new sound.

Moving to the Music

Purpose: Motor imitation and vocal imitation
Items Needed: MP3 player/iPod/CD player; music
Target Group: Babies who are babbling or producing single words

Instructions:
■ Observe your baby as he listens to different baby songs and find one that he enjoys moving to. The song may be part of a collection that you purchased for your MP3 player or one that is routinely played on a children's television show.
■ Imitate your baby's movement (swaying, bouncing) and then add another component such as clapping or marching.

- Encourage him to imitate your movements ("clap, clap, clap").
- Once your child is imitating your movements, add some sounds or words to the routine. For a young baby, you might sing along with the music, replacing the words with a simple syllable you have heard your child say ("la, la, la"). For an older toddler, you might say "dance, dance, dance" or "clap, clap, clap," or simply repeat a word that occurs often in the song.

Sound Associations

Purpose:	Encourage listening, babbling, and imitation
Items Needed:	Toys
Target Group:	Babies who are babbling or producing single words

Instructions:
- Associate different sounds/words with your child's toys to encourage new sound production.

car:	"puhpuhpuh"
eating:	"mmmmm"
smelly diaper:	"eeyew"
sheep:	"baabaa"
kitty:	"meow"
doggy:	"woof-woof"
bee:	"buzzzzz"
snake:	"sssssssss"
baby sleeping:	"shhhhhh"

Daily Routines: Bathing

Purpose:	Word and sound imitation
Items Needed:	Soap, wash cloth, towel, water toys, mesh bag
Target Group:	Babies who are babbling or producing single words

Instructions:
- Place water toys in a bag in which the toys are visible (e.g., net bag).

- Have multiples of several toys (e.g., 2 boats) and toys that begin or end with *m, n, w, p, b, t, d, k, g, f.* When your child is in the tub, have the toy bag visible to the child and wait a few seconds for him to reach for a toy.
- If your child names the toy, repeat the word, emphasizing any sounds in the word that he used incorrectly.
- If your child does not name a toy, say the toy's name, and take it out of the bag.
- Use the toy in water play, modeling action words following your child's lead. Use words to describe your child's actions with the toys (for example, go, push, wash, down, up).
- To encourage your child's participation, take the same toy your child is playing with and imitate his actions with the toy. This often catches your child's attention and provides an opportunity to model words.
- When your child is finished with play, dry each toy with a towel. This gives your child an opportunity to name the toy or use the verb *dry*. Or, if you want to model two-word combinations, you can work on eliciting the name of the object plus the word *dry* (e.g., "dog is dry," "dry the kitty").
- Play a washing game. Wash a body part and model the name. Wait for your child to request more. Use some soap and a washcloth to give baby a bubble bath. Most children enjoy the water activity, and you can add toys to baby's bath to make it fun.

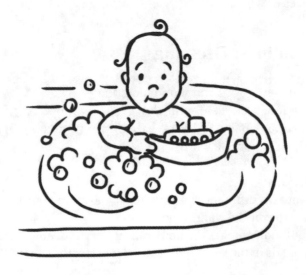

Sample objects and actions:

Objects	Action
Boats	Go, ride
Ball (heavy and light)	Push, up, throw, catch
Baby	Pour, eat, sit, drink
Duck	In, go, bite
Cow	Out, in, eat
Wind up water toys	Wash, wet, dry, go
Cups	In, out, pour, drink, juice, milk, cocoa

Variations:
- Encourage repetitive activities to permit practice with words (e.g., pouring a small quantity of water, and then waiting for your child to ask for more).
- Once your child can produce sounds in single words, use the words in two- or three-word sentences. When your child uses one word at a time, add a word or two to make a simple but complete sentence. Your child may repeat your sentence. This gives him a chance to practice sounds in the longer sequences of words.

Daily Routines: Dressing

> **Purpose:** Word and sound imitation
> **Items Needed:** Clothes for the day
> **Target Group:** Babies who are babbling or producing single words

Instructions:
- Present two different clothing items and have your toddler choose the one he wants to wear.
- If your toddler names the item, repeat the word, emphasizing any sounds in the word that he used incorrectly.

- If your toddler does not name the item, say the name and wait a few seconds to give him time to imitate. If he does not repeat the word, choose an item and give it to him.
- Talk about what you are doing while putting on your child's clothes.
- Provide pauses in your talking to give your child an opportunity to talk.
- Continue to give two options for remaining clothes.

Variations:
- Put clothing items on wrong body part (e.g., socks on hands). Wait for your child to notice and comment.
- Once your child can produce sounds in single words, use the words in short, two- or three-word sentences. Your child may repeat your sentence. This gives him a chance to practice sounds in the longer sequences of words.

Daily Routines: Snack

Purpose:	Word and sound imitation
Items Needed:	Drink and snack items, containers with lids, and a cup
Target Group:	Babies who are babbling or producing single words

Instructions:
- When your child wants a snack, put it in clear containers that are not easy to open and present a cup with a small portion of drink.
- Give your child small portions of food and drink and wait for him to request more. Model "open" or "more." You may take this opportunity to model snack or drink names.
- If your child names the snack, repeat the word, emphasizing any sound in the word that he used incorrectly.
- If your child does not name the snack, model the name and wait a few seconds to let him imitate. If he does not repeat the word, give more snack and repeat the procedure.

Snacks with High Pressure Consonants
Apple
Banana
Cheerios
Cheese
Cookie
Cracker
Carrots
Juice
Popsicle

Variations:
- Have a snack with your child and you request a snack from him.
- Once your child can produce sounds in single words, use the words in two- or three-word sentences. Your child may repeat your sentence. This gives your child a chance to practice sounds in the longer sequences of words.
- By expanding your child's words into a short sentence during the activity, you are encouraging your child to imitate some or all of your sentence. We know that your expansion of your child's words is interpreted by your child as a cue to imitate your expansion. Adult expansions and child imitations are powerful language facilitation techniques

Hide and Seek

Purpose:	Word and sound imitation
Items Needed:	Favorite toys
Target Group:	Babies who are babbling or producing single words

Instructions:
- Hide a toy in an obvious place and encourage your child to find it.

- Each time your child finds the toy, say "yay!" Repeat this activity with different toys, saying "yea" each time your child finds the toy.
- After several turns, let your child find the toy but do not say anything. Your child will expect you to say "yea" and may say it for you when you remain silent.
- Once your baby begins routinely saying "yay" after each toy is found, you can stimulate new words (or short phrases for older toddlers) by labeling each toy when it is found ("ball," "Hi, ball," "Yay...ball!"). Your baby may not be using all the sounds in the word or may be substituting sounds. This is common for young children, but we want you to repeat your baby's word while emphasizing a sound that he did not correctly produce. For example, if your baby says "ma" for "ball," you can repeat "ball" while emphasizing the b. Just this simple modification of the word can help your baby attend to the difference in how the word sounds.

Variations:
- Toddlers love to hide objects, so do not be surprised if your toddler decides to switch roles with you!

Puppet Talk

Purpose:	Word and sound imitation
Items Needed:	Hand puppet, mirror (if available)
Target Group:	Babies who are babbling or producing single words

Instructions:
- Place baby on your lap in front of a mirror (or facing you if no mirror is available).
- Move the puppet's mouth so that it talks to your baby.
- Have the puppet make different sounds/noises and encourage your baby to imitate them. Hold the puppet next to your mouth as you make different sounds.
- Encourage your baby to touch the puppet's mouth as sounds are made. Place your baby's hand on your mouth as you repeat the sounds.

- This is a perfect situation for getting your baby to make lip smacks (kisses), say "aahh" (for hugs), and blow raspberries.
- The transition from babbling to words often happens gradually. Once your baby begins repeating sounds, the next step is for you to model words. Have the puppet perform different actions (e.g., kiss, hug, eat, blow, tickle, night-night) and model words while the puppet performs the action. Keep the play fun for your child. Periodically, wait with the puppet and see if your child tries to use a word. Repeat the word and action and continue playing.

Animal Play

> **Purpose:** Word and sound imitation
> **Items Needed:** Small plastic or stuffed animals
> **Target Group:** Babies babbling or producing single words

Instructions:
- Place different animals in a pillowcase (or other cloth bag).
- Shake the bag and encourage your baby to explore what is inside.
- If your baby does not show an interest in the activity, position an animal so that it is peeking out of the bag.
- Encourage your baby to pull each animal out one at a time. As your baby pulls each animal out, make an appropriate noise to go with each animal.
- Once your baby has removed all of the animals, replace them one at a time saying, "Bye-bye, kitty," "The kitty goes bye-bye," etc.

Animal Noises:

cat	"meow"
dog	"woof"
snake	"sssss"
bird	"caw caw"

Pretend Cooking

Purpose: Word and sound imitation
Items Needed: Play dishes, food items, toy stove (optional)
Target Group: Babies who are producing single words

Instructions:
- Place dishes and food items in a bag or container so the toys are not visible. Have multiples of several toys (e.g., plates, cups, spoons) that begin with *m, n, w, p, b, t, d, k, g, f, s, sh*. Provide an incomplete set of toys (for example, one cup, one bowl, no spoon) to encourage your child to request needed items.
- Present a toy and wait a few seconds for your child to name the toy. Let him select several toys but avoid having him dump all the toys out.
- If your child names the toy, repeat the word, emphasizing the beginning sounds in the word that he used incorrectly. If your child does not name the toy, say the toy name and take it out of the bag.
- If your child does not say the word, prompt with "Say _____." Do not be concerned if your child does not respond at first.
- Set the dishes out for you and your child as your child selects and names them as in a "tea party." Pretend to eat food, making comments such as "I like peas" or "More pizza, please." You can prompt your child to get more toys out of the container by saying, "Can I have more?" or "I'm thirsty."
- Let your child notice whether you have enough food or dishes for the party. Wait for your child to add toys if needed. If your child loses interest in the activity, try to pull more toys out. Discontinue the activity if your child does not resume interest.

Sample Objects/Words:

Objects	Actions/Locations/Descriptors
Plates	Eat, dirty, on
Cups	Drink, milk, pour

Fork	Cut, eat
Knife	Open, cut
Spoon	In, eat
Cookie	On, eat, bite
Cracker	More, eat, bite
Apple	Bite, cut
Banana	Dirty, peel, bite
Carrots	Hot, cut, eat
Juice, milk, cocoa, tea, coffee	Drink, cold, pour, hot

Variations:
- Change the food used in the activity or substitute real food to keep your child's interest.
- Once your child can produce sounds in single words, use the words in two- or three-word sentences. When he uses one word at a time, add a word or two to make a simple sentence. Your child may repeat your sentence. This gives him a chance to practice sounds in the longer sequences of sounds.

Playing with Dolls

> **Purpose:** Word and short phrase imitation
> **Items Needed:** Baby dolls (2), toy beds (2), blankets (2), books (2)
> **Target Group:** Babies who are producing single words

Instructions:
- Place toys in a bag and place the bag in front of your child. Wait for your child to remove one of the toys. If he makes no attempt to do so, peek in the bag and say "look."
- As your child removes each toy, wait for him to name it. If your child names the toy, repeat the word, emphasizing any sounds in the word that he used incorrectly.

- If your child does not name a toy, say the toy name and encourage him to repeat it (even though he may not do so). "Can you say *baby*?"
- Wait for your child to begin playing with the baby doll (either undressing it, reading it a story, or putting it to bed).
- Model your child's actions with the doll using appropriate words to describe what your child is doing (e.g., *night-night, wake-up baby, rock the baby*).
- To encourage your child's participation, take the same toy he is playing with and imitate his actions with the toy. This may attract your child's attention and provide an opportunity to model words.
- When your child loses interest in the activity, hold out the bag and encourage him to put each toy away. This will give your child an opportunity to repeat the words. If he makes no effort to name each toy, say "bye-bye, doll," "The doll goes bye-bye," etc.

Variations:
- Other actions/objects you can use with the doll activity include dressing (shoes, socks, bib), grooming (brushing, combing hair), and feeding (bottle, milk, juice).

Go, Car, Go

Purpose:	Word and word combination imitation
Items Needed:	Toy garage or racetrack, cars (2), trucks (2), people to go into cars (multiple), other vehicles (e.g., motorcycle, bike)
Target Group:	Babies/toddlers who are producing words

Instructions:
- Place the toy garage or racetrack in front of your child. If you have a folding garage or racetrack, place it unopened in front of your child.
- Put the other vehicles, people, and props into a bag that your child cannot see through.

- Wait to see if your child requests that you open the garage. If he does not request, open the garage and close it again, saying "open" and "close" while performing the actions.
- If your child does not request that you open the garage with a gesture or vocalization, provide a model by saying "open." Prompt him to say "open." When you obtain some type of response, either pointing to the toy or saying "open" or another appropriate response, repeat what your child says (e.g., "open") and then expand (e.g., "open the garage"). You can emphasize any sounds that your baby does not produce correctly.
- Shake the bag of toys with the props and say, "What do we need to go with the garage?" If he asks for the toys, pull each out of the bag as he asks for them. Otherwise, take two out of the bag, show him both, and ask "Do you want truck or car?" Give him an opportunity to label the object, and if he does not, label the object for him. Then ask him to label the object (e.g., "Can you say *car*?"). Do this until all of the objects have been removed from the bag.
- Next, play with the garage and objects in appropriate ways, describing your child's actions and your own. If your child produces words relating to the activity (child says "car"), first imitate (e.g., "car") and then expand (e.g., "The car is going fast"). If your child does not produce the words on his own, provide a model and ask him to label the object (e.g., "What is this?"). If he is able to label the object, you might try to elicit two-word utterances (e.g., "go car").
- Remember to emphasize sounds that you child does not produce correctly or deletes.

Bouncing Balls

Purpose:	Word and word combination imitation
Items Needed:	Balls of different sizes, containers, basketball hoop
Target Group:	Babies/toddlers who are producing words

Instructions:
- There are lots of activities that can be performed with a ball, such as bouncing, rolling, throwing, patting, dropping. As with

all the activities described in this book, you want to play with your child using the toys described here.

▪ Begin with an activity that is of interest to your child (e.g., roll the ball back and forth, throw the ball into a container, climb on a big exercise ball, etc.). During the activity, provide many opportunities for your child to request and label the ball as well as to do the actions that can be performed with the ball.

▪ You can also emphasize that idea of turn taking. A common activity would be rolling the ball back and forth with your child. You can begin by rolling the ball and saying, "The ball is rolling" or "Roll the ball." When it is your child's turn to roll the ball, say "Your turn. What are you doing?" If he provides the appropriate response, "roll," expand to "yes, roll the ball." If he does not respond, provide the model and a request to repeat it if your child does not do so spontaneously. When you have the ball from that point on, say "my turn" and require your child to ask you to "roll" in response to your question "What do you want me to do?" Or say, "What do you want?" to elicit "ball" instead of roll.

Variations:

▪ Instead of rolling the ball, throw the ball in a container or bounce the ball back and forth with your baby.

▪ Instead of obtaining a one-word response from your child, elicit two words ("roll ball," "bounce ball," "more ball") or three-word utterances (e.g., "Mommy roll ball").

Blowing Party Horns

> **Purpose:** To teach the concept of oral vs. nasal airflow
> **Items Needed:** Simple party horns
> **Target Group:** Toddlers with repaired cleft palate who are purposefully snorting air through the nose during consonant production

Instructions:

- Show your child a party horn and blow it gently. Demonstrate this several times before giving your child a horn to blow.

- Give your child a party horn and ask him to blow. If the horn produces sound, praise your child and say, "Good, the air came out of your mouth." If the sound produced by the horn is weak or if your child blows air through his nose, gently pinch his nostrils together to redirect the air through his mouth and ask him to blow again. Repeat this several times while keeping his nostrils closed. "Good, the air is coming through your mouth!" Then, place your fingers on either side of his nose without pinching the nostrils together and ask him to blow the horn again.

- If air continues to pass through his nose over time, discontinue the activity. Although there are a number of reasons why a child may be unsuccessful blowing a party horn (see discussion below), you do not want to continue an activity of this kind when failure has repeatedly occurred. Failure could be related to VPI. If so, you do not want to repeatedly ask your child to do something he is not physically capable of doing.

Comments:

- Simple party horns can be purchased at most discount stores. Look for horns other than the common birthday party horn (it can be more difficult to blow than other horns). Flute party horns are usually easier to blow.

- A child's ability to blow horns is related to his age, his experience with the task, and his ability to achieve velopharyngeal closure. A twelve-month-old (with or without a cleft) who is asked to blow a horn will probably not know what "blow" means. We typically use this activity with children twenty-four months of age and older, but some eighteen-month-old toddlers may be able to do it as well. If your child has never blown horns before, it may take him a while to get the idea of blowing.

■ Since most children with repaired cleft palate have the physical ability to achieve velopharyngeal closure, they will respond quickly to this activity once they understand what blowing is and have some time to practice with a party horn. Children with VPI may or may not be able to blow these horns without pinching their nostrils together. If your child is unable to do this activity over time without his nostrils pinched shut, discontinue it and focus on activities designed to increase your child's language and speech sound skills.

■ Once your child can direct air through the mouth to blow a horn repeatedly, there is no need to continue the activity (unless, of course, your child just wants to play with the horns). Move on to speech activities so that your child begins associating oral airflow with speech.

■ Some horns have small parts and represent a potential choking hazard, so adult supervision of this activity is required!

Follow-up activity:
■ See Bug Race below.

Bug Race!

Purpose:	To stimulate oral airflow for consonants
Items Needed:	Ball, table (or other hard surface), pom-pom bugs
Target Group:	Toddlers who are producing words but not yet producing high-pressure consonants (this activity stimulates *p*)

Instructions:
■ Create two bugs—one for you and one for your child—by attaching self-adhesive wiggle eyes (use felt eyes for very young toddlers) on a pom-pom. These materials can be found in most craft stores.

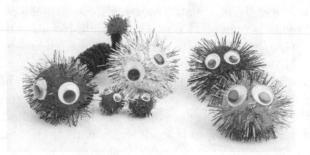

- Put the bug on a table. Place your chin on the table with your lips approximately two inches from the bug. Produce a raspberry ("ppppppp") to move it across the table.
- Your child will likely laugh as the cotton ball flies across the table and will try to do it too.
- For older children, line both bugs up side by side and have a bug race!

Comments:
- *Do not blow* the bug across the table or allow your child to do so. The purpose of this activity is to build up pressure behind the lips for *p*. Produce a raspberry, and if your child does not imitate you, ask him to "spit" the bug across the table. Demonstrate by making an explosive *p*.
- If your child is unable to produce a raspberry because of air loss through the nose, gently pinch his nostrils closed and ask him to do it again. Repeat this process several times. Then, place your fingers on the side of your child's nose but do not close off the nostrils. As your child produces a raspberry during this trial, determine if oral airflow occurred (some air is passing through the mouth if "pppppp" is heard). Discontinue the activity if your child is unable to do it after repeated trials.
- The bugs are small and represent a potential choking hazard, so adult supervision of this activity is required!

Variations:
- Use a cotton ball or ping pong ball if pom-poms are not available.
- Or, hold a tissue in front of your mouth and say "puh" to make it move. Remember, no blowing!

Follow-up Activity:
▪ Once your child successfully produces a raspberry (prolonged *p*) to move the bug across the table, introduce activities that will give your child the opportunity to use oral airflow to put the *p* in words. For example, blow bubbles and ask your child to pop them. Each time he pops a bubble, say "pop, pop, pop!"

8

Velopharyngeal Inadequacy (VPI)

Velopharyngeal clo-sure is an important term that has been referred to throughout this book. Recall from Chapter 1 that velopharyngeal closure occurs when the soft palate moves up and back against the back wall of the throat during speech. This action effectively separates the nose from the mouth and is required for production of all consonants in English except the three nasal consonants—*m, n, ng* (as in the word si<u>ng</u>). Air must be allowed to pass into the nose in order to achieve the nasal quality needed for these three consonants.

When the soft palate is unable to reach the back wall of a person's throat to seal off the nose (either because the palate is too short or does not move well), velopharyngeal inadequacy (VPI) occurs. VPI results in the opposite problem from what occurs when you have a cold and are congested. Whereas nasal congestion leads to speech that sounds *hypo-nasal* (not enough air is resonating in the nose during nasal consonants), VPI leads to speech that sounds *hypernasal* (too much air is resonating in the nose at inappropriate times). When a child's hypernasality is se-vere enough to call attention to her speech or prevents her from being understood, surgery is typically recommended.

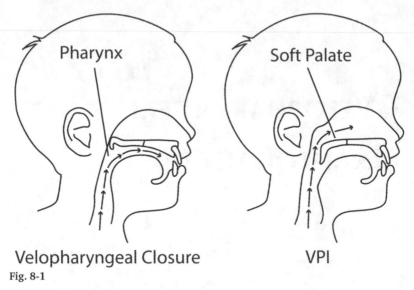

Velopharyngeal Closure   **VPI**

Fig. 8-1

In addition to causing hypernasality, which is heard primarily on vowels, VPI often results in nasal airflow, which is heard on pressure consonants as well. This is known as *audible nasal emission*. We produce pressure consonants by creating constrictions in the mouth (such as pressing the lips together for *p*, lifting the tongue tip up to the hard palate for *s*, lifting the back of the tongue up for *k*, etc.). For English speakers, air pressure builds up behind the constriction to produce either an explosive sound (such as *p, b, t, d, k*, and *g*) or a noisy sound (such as *f, s, z*, and *sh*). When a child has VPI, however, air pressure that should be building up behind the constriction in her mouth is compromised by air leaking into the nose. Once the child with VPI releases the constriction, some air may flow from her mouth. This may result in the production of an identifiable consonant, but air is also flowing through the child's nose and may create an audible snorting quality.

Although hypernasality and audible nasal emission distort speech, they rarely interfere with a listener's ability to understand the child's speech if she uses correct lip and tongue placement when speaking. This distinction becomes important when treatment decisions are being made and will be further discussed below.

Before a baby's palate is surgically repaired, the cleft prevents separation of the nose and mouth. Consequently, you might expect that your baby's babbling might sound hypernasal before her CP is repaired. In reality, however, hypernasality is not frequently noticed in babbling.

We usually do not hear a distinctly nasal quality until after a baby's palate has been repaired and she has begun to talk. If VPI is present, then hypernasality will be increasingly obvious as a child begins combining words into sentences. Remember, though, only an estimated 20 percent of children with a repaired CP have difficulty achieving velopharyngeal closure.

∷ Why Does VPI Occur?

Many children with repaired CP have a soft palate that is too short to achieve velopharyngeal closure. Other children have a palate that is long enough but does not move well. These two types of problems reflect either a structural or neurological problem, so they can only be treated surgically (or with a prosthetic device when surgery is not an option). Speech therapy cannot fix VPI when it is related to a physical problem.

∷ What Is "Learned" or Phoneme-Specific VPI?

Occasionally, children with repaired CP learn to produce specific consonants (usually *s,* but sometimes *z, sh, ch,* and *j*), with air passing through the nose. Because they produce all other sounds correctly without evidence of hypernasality or inappropriate nasal air flow, we know that these children are capable of achieving velopharyngeal closure. This problem is called "phoneme-specific" or "sound-specific" VPI and represents a learned behavior. We do not know why some children learn to produce specific sounds with the velopharyngeal port open, but the problem is easily corrected with speech therapy.

∷ How Is VPI Diagnosed?

The first indication that a child may have VPI comes from her speech. If she sounds hypernasal and has audible nasal emission, the adequacy of the velopharyngeal mechanism for speech will be questioned.

If your child's speech sounds excessively nasal, the SLP on her cleft palate team will perform a speech evaluation to determine the most likely cause: 1) VPI, 2) a palatal fistula, or 3) simply mislearning how to produce certain speech sounds. If VPI is suspected, she will be referred for either an endoscopic assessment or an x-ray study (video-fluoroscopy). Some institutions recommend both.

An endoscopic assessment involves placing a small fiber-optic scope (tube) in the child's nose and observing the velopharyngeal mechanism while she talks. Many centers numb the nose (with a spray solution) before placing the scope so that the child is comfortable with the scope in place. Endoscopes can be very long, and the length of the scope can be scary to a young child, even though only a couple of inches of the scope is actually placed in the nose. Nasoendoscopy is typically recommended for children who are old enough to cooperate with the procedure—approximately four years of age and older. Cooperation involves not only tolerating the scope in the nose (without crying) but repeating a speech sample as well.

Many SLPs and surgeons prefer to do nasoendoscopy rather than an x-ray study because all of the velopharyngeal structures can be viewed at the same time as they move during speech and because the image is more easily interpreted. In contrast, a comprehensive x-ray study may require several different images to provide the same information. Although some centers will recommend either procedure, many only recommend an x-ray study if a child will not cooperate for nasoendoscopy. Figure 8-2 shows an image seen on nasoendoscopy.

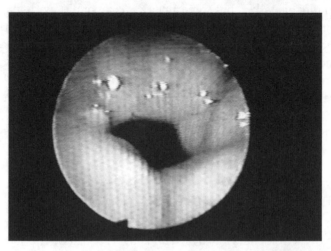

Fig. 8-2. *View of velopharyngeal structures seen on nasoendoscopy. At the top of the image is the back wall of the throat (which has moved forward). At the bottom of the image is the soft palate (which has elevated and moved toward the back wall of the throat). VPI is evident by the large central gap (hole).*

▪▪ When Is a Formal Diagnosis of VPI Made?

In our experience, there is probably no problem more frustrating to parents and SLPs than having to delay a formal diagnosis of VPI when a child's speech sounds excessively nasal. Even if VPI is suspected in a young toddler, a formal assessment will usually not be made until your child is three or four years old. There are several reasons:

- *The child must be old enough to cooperate during the assessment and repeat specific words that she is asked to say.* As explained above, the procedures used to evaluate the velopharyngeal mechanism, including nasoendoscopy and videofluoroscopy (an x-ray procedure), are often scary for a very young child and it may be difficult for the child to cooperate for them. In such cases, when the child is receiving speech therapy, the SLP may focus on improving articulation and ignore nasality until a formal assessment of VPI can be performed.

- *Before a child's ability to achieve velopharyngeal closure can be evaluated, she must be producing some high-pressure consonants that require velopharyngeal closure* (such as p, b, t, d, k, g, f, v, s, z, sh, ch). If your child is not trying to produce some of these sounds, then it is not possible to evaluate the *potential* of her velopharyngeal mechanism to achieve closure. For example, we may hear early signs of VPI (such as hypernasality) in a two-year-old child, but if her consonant development is not age appropriate, we may not be able to interpret the significance of the "nasal" sounding speech.

  Consider a child who only produces five consonants, such as w, y, m, n, h. This child is not producing the pressure consonants that require tight velopharyngeal closure (such as the stops and fricatives described earlier), and so she frequently substitutes nasal consonants (m and n) for those consonants in words. The child's speech is not understood (because she is using the wrong consonant) and sounds very nasal (because many of the target consonants in words are being substituted with a nasal consonant). We cannot accurately diagnose VPI in such children because they are making *no attempt* to produce sounds that require velopharyngeal closure. These children need speech therapy to help them expand their repertoire of consonants so that we can hear (and see) what happens when they attempt to produce the correct sound.

■ *The clinical significance of mild hypernasality may be questioned.* Some children produce a large variety of consonants (including pressure consonants), but their speech is not easily understood because they do not use the consonants appropriately in conversation. When these children have mild hypernasality, we wait until their articulation improves and their speech is more easily understood before making a decision to pursue (or not) a formal assessment of velopharyngeal function.

If an imaging study confirms that a child has VPI, the information on the nasoendoscopic tape or x-ray is used to identify the best treatment option. As discussed in Chapter 5, there are several surgical procedures that can be performed to treat VPI. Your child's surgeon will determine which option is best for your child.

❚❚ Conclusion

As you can see, an accurate diagnosis of VPI may be a quick, straightforward process for some children but a drawn-out, complicated affair for others. If your child's cleft palate team suspects VPI but is not recommending surgery, make sure that you understand why. Our goal is to ensure that, whenever possible, VPI is resolved before a child begins school. Although we can all probably agree that providing treatment sooner is better than later, there are some valid reasons why VPI cannot always be treated as soon as it is discovered.

9

SPECIAL CONCERNS IF YOUR CHILD WAS INTERNATIONALLY ADOPTED

If you adopted a child with a cleft palate (CP) from outside of the United States or Canada, you and your child may face special challenges. These challenges may result from less-than-ideal treatment (or no treatment) for CP and other medical conditions prior to adoption, lack of speech therapy at an early age, or a number of other factors related to your child's early care. Although these difficulties may make it more of a challenge for your child to "catch up" to children with clefts who have received optimal care since birth, the obstacles are by no means insurmountable. With your help, your child can make tremendous progress with early treatment.

The team care for these children is different from those who are receiving traditional follow-up care from a cleft palate team. The children begin their team care later, and that care can be complicated by previous medical and surgical treatment and an uncertain social history. These children are reported to be at risk for speech-language and developmental delays related to a variety of prenatal, birth, and early developmental factors stemming from the situation surrounding their adoptive history. These factors (listed below) may individually or in combination influence development even after adoption.

:: Medical and Developmental Factors That Can Affect Development

- maternal and early infant nutritional deficiencies
- unknown birth complications
- poor health care
- issues related to learning a second language
- age of adoption
- presence of associated genetic conditions
- lack of hearing monitoring or follow-up
- late or no surgical cleft lip and/or palate repairs

In 2014, 6,441 children were adopted in the United States from 99 different countries, with the majority coming from China, Ethiopia, and Haiti. Internationally adopted (IA) children often present unique challenges to professionals on cleft palate teams. Some reports suggest that these children are more likely than nonadopted children to have more severe clefts (such as bilateral cleft lip and palate) and to be carriers of antibiotic resistant bacteria (Hansson et al., 2012; Sullivan, Jung, & Mulliken, 2014). Both of these factors can complicate your child's treatment and influence outcomes. The treatment plan developed by your child's team may also differ from a typical treatment plan because age at time of the adoption can influence the priorities for and timing of surgery. For example, lip surgery is typically performed before palatal surgery in the United States. But some surgeons opt to repair the palate first for a child with an unrepaired CLP if the child is older when he is adopted to promote speech and language development (Sullivan et al., 2014; Hansson et al., 2012).

Even when a child's lip and palate are repaired before he comes to his adoptive country, these operations are frequently performed later than is typical in North America and European countries. The later that a CP is successfully repaired, the more likely your child will have persistent delays in speech and language development.

Studies of adopted children with CP have reported higher rates of VPI and palatal fistula following palatal surgery, and these children typically require more surgeries to improve their speech (Sullivan et al., 2014). Some surgeons believe these children are more challenging to treat because they are older when they finally have surgery (Hansson et al., 2012; Sullivan et al., 2014).

▪▪ Adoptions of Children with Cleft Lips Are on the Upswing

Recently, the overall number of children adopted internationally into the United States and Europe has fallen. But cleft palate teams report that the numbers of children with clefts who were adopted internationally (IA) has actually increased (Hansson, Svensson, & Becker, 2012; Swanson, Smartt, Salzman, Brigfeld, Hopper, Gruss, & Tse, 2014). In fact, a report from a large cleft palate-craniofacial team found that the number of internationally adopted children has increased five-fold and now accounts for 12 percent of their patients with cleft lip and/or palate (Swanson, et al., 2014). In one study, 80 percent of the IA children with cleft lip and/or cleft palate were adopted from China.

▪▪ Early Development of Children Adopted Internationally

Many studies have been done on the early development of internationally adopted children. But the vast majority of children in these studies did not have clefts. For any given adopted child, all of the factors listed above could affect language development. But the current evidence suggests that most young children adopted internationally progress rapidly in learning their new language and make good progress at school.

When children with clefts are adopted during the infant/toddler period, they learn language rapidly (Tan & Yang, 2005). In fact, studies have reported that IA infants and toddlers may completely catch up after living with their adoptive families for an average of sixteen months (Tan & Yang, 2005; Glennen, 2007, 2008, 2014; Snedeker, et al., 2007). We know less about children adopted at later ages, but the longer children are in institutional care, the more likely they are to have language or speech delays (Glennen, 2008). The language learning advantage associated with being adopted at a younger age is particularly relevant for children who are adopted from an institutional setting (Roberts et al., 2005).

Prior language experience in the heritage language has no effect on the adopted child's ability to learn a new language (Glennen, 2008). Unlike children who are truly bilingual, most adopted children are only bilingual for a short time during the transition to their second language. Many children lose their heritage (original) language within twenty-two weeks as their skills in the second language improve (Gindis, 2003).

Children who are internationally adopted benefit from early assessment and intervention to reduce the impact of early environmental experiences (Glennen, 2007). Assessment soon after your child joins your family is recommended. The assessment should be provided by a speech-language pathologist (SLP) with experience working with young children with cleft palate. The SLP will describe your child's speech and language development and make recommendations for language learning and, if necessary, early intervention.

An excellent website for information on language development for internationally adopted children is Sharon Glennen's website at http://pages.towson.edu/sglennen/index.htm.

:: Early Development of IA Children with Clefts

The medical histories of IA children are often incomplete or nonexistent, so you may have been told little or nothing about your child's health when you adopted him. However, children with CLP often have had birth complications or early feeding issues that could affect their early development. We know that early nutrition influences growth and development. Studies have shown that adopted children without clefts overcome early nutritional and environmental adversity within two years of adoption (Palacios, Roman, & Camacho, 2014). To date, however, researchers have not studied whether children with clefts also overcome these disadvantages so quickly.

In North America, feeding difficulties in children with CLP are readily resolved, but this may not be the case in your child's country of origin. Feeding and nutrition are among the first issues to be addressed for any child who is adopted. Your child may require consultation with a dietitian or speech-language pathologist to develop a feeding and nutritional plan to maximize his growth. However, considering how well adopted children without clefts do, we would expect your child to make rapid improvement in general growth and development. Your child's cleft palate team will provide resources and referrals for feeding and nutritional issues. As mentioned in Chapter 3, the Cleft Palate Foundation also has feeding resources available for parents at http://www.cleftline.org.

Researchers have found that children without clefts who have been internationally adopted rapidly pick up speech and language skills following adoption. However, there have been few studies of the development of adopted children with CP (Scherer, Kaiser, & Totino, 2012).

One factor that can influence a child's speech, language, and cognitive development in general is his interpersonal interaction. Your child's ability to interact with you and others in his environment will form the foundation for his communicative and intellectual development.

While most internationally adopted children go on to develop good interpersonal skills, a small number of them have behavioral and attention difficulties that require intervention (Miller, 2000; Wilson, 2009). If present, these issues can affect communicative development. In addition, the later age for palate repair for many internationally adopted children results in slower speech development, which further limits early language development.

A small study of ten children (aged eighteen to thirty-six months of age) with clefts (five IA and five nonadopted children) examined language and speech development (Scherer, Kaiser, & Totino, 2012). The researchers found that the internationally adopted children with clefts who had been in the United States at least six months quickly learned to understand English. The IA and nonadopted children with cleft palate performed similarly on cognitive and language comprehension measures, even though the IA group had been in the United States for less than a year. However, the expressive language skills of the IA children—particularly their early vocabulary development—remained behind the nonadopted children's skills. In addition, the speech development of the internationally adopted children was delayed more than we would expect for children with CP born in the United States. The IA children were slower to acquire high-pressure sounds (e.g., *p, b, t, d, k, g, f, v, s, z, ch, sh*), which are particularly problematic for young children with CP. As a result of these differences, the speech of the IA children was more difficult to understand.

Findings from this small pilot study support the need for immediate referral for early speech and language intervention for children with CP who are internationally adopted. These interventions can help minimize the effects of later palate repair and any adverse environmental experiences the children had early in life.

■■ Recommendations for IA Children with CLP

If you have adopted or are in the process of adopting a child with CP, we recommend taking the following steps to help maximize your child's development:

- Immediately contact your local cleft palate team, if you have not already. To find your nearest team, please contact the American Cleft Palate-Craniofacial Association at http://www.cleftline.org/parents-individuals/team-care/.
- Get your child's speech and language development assessed as soon after adoption as possible. Usually these assessments occur within three to six months after a child's arrival in the United States. The assessment will establish a starting point in your child's acquisition of English, identify feeding difficulties that may require intervention, and identify any behavioral problems that may interfere with communicative development. The speech-language pathologist (SLP) on your child's cleft palate team will provide this assessment or refer you to an SLP in your area.
- Make sure your child receives comprehensive assessments from the cleft palate team to identify any medical or developmental issues that should be addressed. (See Chapter 2.)
- If your child is aged two or younger, enroll him in an early intervention program that provides speech and language intervention with parent training. (See Chapter 6.)
- If your child is three or older, contact your local school system for information about special education services, including speech and language therapy, that your child may be eligible for.

10
LOOKING FORWARD...
SOME FINAL
THOUGHTS

Earlier chapters focused mainly on concerns of babies and toddlers with cleft lip and palate (CLP), with special emphasis on strategies that can be used to promote good speech and language development. Although some toddlers with clefts do not need formal early intervention services, we are strong advocates for those services when delays are identified. We firmly believe that addressing problems early on can minimize the severity of problems seen later.

For some children with cleft palate (CP), early intervention may be all that is needed. But other children need additional treatment (including surgery and speech-language therapy) during the preschool and school-aged years. This chapter provides an overview of the speech problems and other issues that older children with clefts sometimes have.

■■ Your Child's Speech

The speech and language skills your child develops early in life serve as an important foundation for her later speech and language

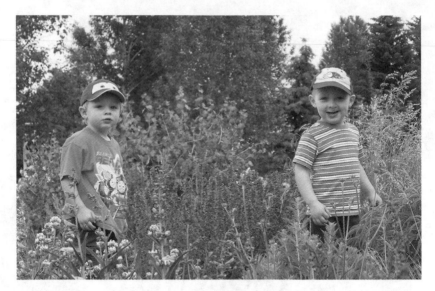

development. Research has shown that there is an association between early speech-language behaviors (such as how frequently a baby vocalizes and the diversity of consonants she uses when babbling) and later performance. Thus, early intervention can be thought of as an important investment you make in your child.

Some children who receive early intervention do not need the formal services of a speech-language pathologist (SLP) once they enter the preschool years, but many do. Our focus in early intervention for young children is to enhance language development and increase the number of different consonants they can produce. Once a child enters the preschool years, the focus of therapy often expands. We do not just want to ensure that the child can produce age-appropriate consonants. We also want to help her put consonants together to produce speech that is easily understood.

As discussed in Chapter 6, toddlers learning to talk are often faced with a dilemma. Some words they want to use contain consonants or consonant combinations that are just difficult to say. A fifteen-month-old toddler might solve this problem by saying only easy words. As children get older, though, it becomes increasingly hard for them to avoid saying difficult words. The typical two-year-old might solve this problem by omitting final consonants in some words ("wa-" for *watch*), leaving off syllables in long words ("te-phone" for *telephone*), and omitting one consonant in a consonant blend ("bu" for *blue*). The child may also begin to substitute easier sounds (*m, n, b, p, t, d, w*) for harder sounds (*k, g, s, z, sh, ch, y, r, l*). So, while a toddler under three years of age will delete many consonants to make pronunciation easier, by the time she is three, she will mostly use substitution errors for difficult words.

Preschoolers whose speech is developing normally make a number of such sound substitutions. These substitutions simplify speech for young children as their language and motor skills are maturing and should slowly disappear as they get older. When preschoolers are difficult to understand, it is usually due to one of two reasons. First, they may only produce a small number of consonants, which they must use to produce a large number of different words in their vocabulary. Second, they are using the typical sound omissions and substitutions that all preschoolers use during normal speech-language development, but these substitutions are simply persisting longer than they should.

When sound substitutions are part of the normal developmental process and are appropriate for a child's age, listeners can usually figure out what the child is saying. For example, most of us understand that a three-year-old who says "wabbit" intends to say "rabbit." When sound substitutions persist beyond a certain age or when a sound substitution is unusual ("tabbit" for "rabbit"), a child's speech intelligibility is usually affected.

An SLP will consider many factors (such as when a child began to talk, how difficult the child is to understand, and how unusual

‖ Speech Intelligibility

Speech intelligibility refers to how easily an individual's speech can be understood. A child does not have to correctly say all sounds in a word for it to be intelligible. For example, a two-year-old child might point to a dog and say "goggy." The pronunciation of the word may not be totally accurate, but adults know that the child is saying "doggy." As a general rule of thumb, approximately 75 percent of everything a three-year-old child says should be understood by a stranger. That percentage should increase to 90 percent for a four-year-old child. If your child's speech is not easily understood, a speech-language pathologist can evaluate her to determine whether she would benefit from therapy.

the sound substitutions are) when deciding whether direct speech therapy is needed. Your input is important to this process. So, keep a diary of the words your child says incorrectly, including examples of how each word is said, and take that list to your child's SLP or to a speech-language evaluation. Also, remember that if your child does not qualify for speech-language therapy services at school, and your insurance is not willing to pay for private therapy, you have the option of paying for it privately.

VPI

A key responsibility of the SLP on the cleft palate team is to monitor your child's speech for evidence of VPI (including hypernasality and audible nasal emission) during the preschool years. Ideally, the diagnosis of VPI will be made for most children by the time they are four or five years old. This ensures that any surgery needed for the problem can be carried out before the child goes to school.

That said, we must admit that the decision to refer a child for surgery can sometimes be difficult to make. When a child's speech consistently has severe hypernasality and audible nasal emission, we feel comfortable in supporting a surgical recommendation. Some children, however, may have mild hypernasality without nasal emission. If that same child has severe articulation problems, we may take a more cautious approach and recommend reevaluation of her nasality once her articulation errors have been eliminated or substantially reduced. Why? Because the mild hypernasality may not seem as significant once the child's speech is more easily understood. (Of course, the reverse is true, too—the child's hypernasality may sound worse.)

As SLPs, we know that listeners (us included!) sometimes have difficulty separating the effects of articulation from those of nasality. When we listen to a child who has poor speech intelligibility, our first instinct may be to quickly treat whatever we can to improve the child's speech. The problem is that eliminating mild hypernasality with surgery will not make an unintelligible child easier to understand. If your child has hypernasality and the SLP or other members of the cleft palate team are dragging their feet when it comes to diagnosing or treating VPI, discuss your concerns with them. They should be able to provide you with a good reason for the delay.

■ Some SLPs Believe...

- *Teaching a child to produce speech sounds is easier when VPI has been surgically corrected.* At this time, we know of no research that supports this claim. We can say with confidence that children with obvious VPI can learn to correctly produce their error sounds in speech therapy. We routinely recommend speech therapy to teach preschoolers correct articulation, and we advise SLPs and parents to simply ignore any hypernasality and audible nasal until an assessment of the child's velopharyngeal mechanism can be carried out (see Chapter 8).
- *The presence of VPI, regardless of severity, justifies a recommendation for surgery.* We do not agree with this philosophy. Varying degrees of hypernasality are acceptable in different dialects across the country. How much nasality is acceptable? It depends on where you live. We believe that hypernasality (without accompanying audible nasal emission) should only be treated surgically when it is pronounced enough to call negative attention to a child's speech.

Your Child's Dentition

When a preschooler is enrolled in direct speech therapy because of problems with speech intelligibility, our goal is to eliminate errors that result in either the omission of a consonant or the substitution of one consonant for another in a word. These types of errors are considered priorities precisely because they influence how well a child is understood. Typically, we are less concerned about how a child's dentition affects his consonant production at this age. But after the child enters school and substitution/omission errors have (hopefully) resolved, the impact of dentition on speech is considered.

A child's dentition can significantly affect the precision with which she produces the fricative consonants of our language. During normal speech production, "fricative" noise (like the sounds heard when you say "ssss" or "ffff") is produced when air moving through your mouth is channeled through a small space. When teeth are not in their proper position, fricative noise may be created, but the airstream is misdirected so the sound that is produced is distorted.

Fricative Consonants	Example
th (voiceless)	<u>th</u>anks
th (voiced)	fa<u>th</u>er
f	<u>f</u>unny
v	<u>v</u>an
s	<u>s</u>un
z	<u>z</u>oo
sh	<u>sh</u>oe
zh	mea<u>s</u>ure
h	<u>h</u>ouse

Several of these fricatives, including *s, z, sh,* and *zh,* are particularly sensitive to problems with dentition. We produce these four fricatives by using our tongue to direct air toward the biting edge of our front teeth. When teeth are misaligned or do not meet properly along their biting edge, sound distortion can occur.

When a child is born with a cleft that extends through the gum ridge, problems with dentition *may* affect her ability to produce fricative consonants. It is important to point out, though, that some children with misaligned teeth have normal speech, while some children with normal dentition distort certain consonants in their speech.

Your child's SLP will determine whether significant consonant distortion is present, and, if so, whether to initiate treatment or delay it until dental treatment has been completed (see Chapter 5). We have successfully eliminated consonant distortion in some children prior to orthodontic treatment and have had to delay therapy for many others until treatment was complete. When it comes to dentition and its relationship to speech, one size definitely does not fit all!

❚❚ A Word about Your Role and Your Child's Role in the Treatment Process

Your role in the treatment process is a critical one that may change over time. As explained in Chapter 7, your child may qualify for early intervention through your state or county. If so, an Individualized Family Service Plan (IFSP) will be developed for her, specifying what services she will receive and goals for development in areas such as speech and language. Early intervention usually requires parents to actively participate in therapy sessions with an SLP or other therapists and educators. Parents also need to be involved in carrying out the goals of treatment in their child's daily routine.

Once your child begins attending school, you will no longer be present for her speech-language therapy sessions (unless you are paying for private therapy). You may therefore feel less connected to the whole process. If your child qualifies for special education services due to a speech and language delay, an Individualized Education Program (IEP) will be developed for her. The IEP will identify her therapy goals, and meetings will be scheduled periodically to assess her progress. Make sure that you attend those meetings so that you can advocate for your child and update the educational team regarding any surgeries that are planned.

It will be important for you to stay in touch with the SLP throughout the school year so that you know how often your child is receiving therapy, what she is working on in therapy, and how the SLP is evaluating her progress. Remember that you are the link between your child's cleft palate team and her SLP in the public schools. Many team SLPs are willing to contact other SLPs working with children to assist in planning treatment, but parents need to request that contact.

Your child's SLP can also help you identify ways to work on your child's speech-language therapy goals during routine tasks throughout your day. As your child gets older, you may need to carve out ten to fifteen minutes a day to help her with speech. You cannot rely solely on visits to the SLP to correct your child's speech problems. Remember—if your child is enrolled in direct speech therapy at school, she will only be spending approximately one hour per week with an SLP. Although your child will learn how to correctly produce target sounds, she must use what she has learned every day throughout the day in order for the new speech patterns to become habitual. If no one works on your child's speech outside the therapy room, having an SLP work with her on speech once or twice a week for thirty minutes will be of limited benefit to her.

If your child's progress in speech therapy is slow, you can advocate for additional therapy during your child's IEP meeting. If the school cannot provide additional therapy time, ask the team SLP about other speech-language therapy services in your area that might be available to supplement your child's therapy time.

As your child's advocate, it is very important that you see yourself as an active participant in her care. When she has an appointment with the cleft palate team, ask questions...and continue to ask them if you do not understand what you have been told. If you do not like the answers you are receiving, please get a second opinion. We are making a point to say this here because over the years we have heard from parents who were concerned that specific members of their child's team had not taken the time to help them understand recommended treatments. In some cases, these parents proceeded with the treatment even though they did not always understand why it was needed. Any professional who has the time to treat your child should have the time to explain the treatment so that you understand what will be done and why it is needed.

As your child enters the teenage years, it may be appropriate to include her in these treatment discussions as well. Whether the issue is speech or facial appearance, professionals are always asking, "Can I make it better?" The answer may be "yes," but that alone doesn't necessarily mean that treatment should be carried out. Should a teenager's lip be surgically revised just because a surgeon says, "I can make that look better"? Should a teenager be enrolled in speech therapy just because an SLP says her speech can be improved?

No one answer is appropriate for all teenagers and their families. The answer for most teens will be dictated by the value they place on the expected results. If no one reacts negatively to their speech and they are satisfied with their appearance, they may decide that the potential benefits of additional speech therapy or surgery are not worth the costs involved both in terms of time and money. Since we want young people with clefts to be fully informed before making a decision with their parents, we encourage you to give your child the opportunity to discuss treatment recommendations with the professionals involved in her care.

▪▪ Your Child's Changing Perspective

Your child's interest in her speech and physical appearance will undoubtedly change over time. Many preschoolers, with and without clefts, simply don't care about their speech and the difficulties that others may have in understanding them. Others become quickly frustrated when parents and friends do not understand them. That frustration can lead to behavioral problems such as tantrums or reluctance to engage in conversation. As children get older and their speech improves, tantrums typically diminish, but some children may remain reluctant to actively engage others in conversation. These children and adolescents will respond when others ask questions but may not initiate conversation on their own. If you notice that your child is reluctant to talk around others, be sure to talk to her SLP about it.

If your child was born with a cleft involving the lip, the day will come when other children will ask her about it...and adults may ask you about it as well. Although such curiosity is normal, it can be difficult to respond unless you have thought about what you want to say. We believe that a young child who has been given a simple explanation about her cleft is better prepared to address the questions (or teasing) that come her way.

You will want to keep your explanation very simple for a preschool child (for example, "You were born with a hole in your lip"). As she gets older, however, you will need to provide your child with more details about her condition.

In its publication entitled *Preparing Your Child for Social Situations*, the Cleft Palate Foundation makes two important points. The first is that children learn how to respond to questions about their clefts by listening to their parents respond to such questions. If you are not comfortable responding to questions, your child will note this. Make sure you think about how you want to respond to such questions before they arise so that you can provide a simple, forthright explanation.

The second point is that older children getting ready to attend school should be given the correct vocabulary related to clefts so that they can confidently answer questions about their condition. When asked what happened to her lip, a young child might say, "I was born with a hole in my lip, and the doctor fixed it when I was a baby." As she gets older and learns more about her condition, she should be able to provide a more educational response. For example: "I was born with a cleft of the lip. It happened because portions of my lip did not come together properly when my mother was pregnant with me. After I was born, I had surgery to fix it." Being prepared can help children feel more comfortable when confronted with personal questions.

Teasing is a major concern for most parents. As parents ourselves, we know firsthand how cruel young children can be to one another. Teasing is particularly frustrating because it is something our children will encounter that is, for the most part, beyond our control. Although you may not be able to shield your child from teasing, you can do the following:

1. Listen to her concerns.
2. Help her understand that all children get teased for many different reasons.
3. Jointly identify some simple ways for her to respond (see resources on bullying in Resources).

It may also be helpful to seek out opportunities for your child to get together with other children and teens who have clefts. There are a number of summer camps that have been developed specifically for children with a facial difference. These camp experiences can be very uplifting for children because they realize firsthand that they are not alone—that there are others out there with similar problems who are experiencing similar feelings. Sharing these feelings and working through them together can be a very rewarding experience for your child. In addition to offering the same types of fun activities associated with any summer camp, many of these camps have activities that focus on building self-esteem, and some help teens address practical concerns, such as how to apply make-up to minimize the appearance of scars. The Cleft Palate Foundation has a list of some of the camps available in the United States and Canada. Consult with your child's cleft palate team to identify others in your area.

As your child moves into the teenage years, remember that this is a fragile time for all young people. Appearance is a major concern for teens, and the presence of a cleft lip may (or may not) exacerbate your child's concerns about her appearance. It is important that you support your teen by acknowledging (not dismissing) her concerns and then identifying resources that can help her cope with or address them. Some children need only a strong group of friends for support. Others benefit from interacting with other teens who have a cleft and are experiencing similar concerns. Listen to your child. If you are not sure how to help her deal with her feelings about her appearance or with teasing, discuss your concerns with an appropriate professional on her cleft palate team. Your team can refer you to a psychologist (if one is not active on the team itself) who can provide the guidance you need.

Finally, it is important to point out that while there may be some stressful times ahead, they will pass. Rest assured, there is every reason to believe that your child will develop into a confident, resilient adult. Cleft lip and palate will always be part of her life, but it does not have to define who she is. There are many successful adults with clefts in almost any profession you can name who enjoy strong personal relationships and richly rewarding lives.

▪▪ A Final Thought

One final thought to leave you with. Much of what we have written in this book is based on what we have learned over many years of carrying out clinical research studies to better understand how a cleft palate influences speech and language development and how best to evaluate and treat speech and language problems when they occur. We owe a huge debt to the children (and their parents) who participated in our clinical studies.

The parents were not only willing to give freely of their time, but they allowed us the opportunity to get to know them and their children. Some of them we only met once, but others we saw for more extended periods as they participated in intervention studies that lasted several months or in longitudinal studies of speech and language development that sometimes lasted as long as four and a half years. The children did not benefit directly from the information that we gained from those studies, but what we learned from them has affected the way that we view early speech and language development and early intervention for young children with cleft palate today.

Although we have come a long way in understanding and treating the speech and language problems of children with cleft palate, there are still unanswered questions that should be addressed. If professionals on your child's cleft palate team invite your child to participate in their ongoing clinical investigations, we hope you will "pay it forward" and agree to do so. Working together in this way, we can improve the outcomes for children with cleft lip and palate everywhere.

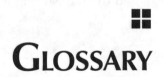

GLOSSARY

Adenoid: a small mass of lymphoid tissue located in the back of the nose on the back wall of the throat. Although adenoids are considered part of the immune system that fights infection, enlarged adenoids may be removed when they interfere with breathing or block the Eustachian tube (which can lead to chronic ear infections).

Alphabet knowledge: knowing about the letters of the alphabet.

Alveolar ridge: the portion of the upper and lower jaw that houses teeth; gum ridge.

Articulation: physical production of a speech sound.

Babbling: production of a consonant or vowel together (e.g., *ba*), or a string of consonants and vowels that are often the same (*bababab*a).

Baby signing: teaching signs or gestures to hearing babies as a way of communicating before they develop spoken words.

Bilateral: two sided.

Bilingual: being exposed to and learning (or having learned) two languages.

Cheiloplasty: lip surgery.

Cleft: an opening in the lip and/or palate.

Comprehension: the ability to understand spoken language.

Cooing: early sounds produced by babies when they are happy.

Deciduous teeth: primary (baby) teeth.

Dentition: refers to the teeth that are housed in the dental arch, including primary and/or adult teeth.

Emergent literacy: knowledge and skills that children have about reading before they are actually able to read.

Expansion/expanding: repeating what a child says but adding something to it.

Eustachian tube: the tube that connects the middle ear to the throat in the back of the nose. The tube, which is typically closed, opens periodically to equalize the pressure in the middle ear with the pressure outside the ears and also assists with drainage of fluid.

Fistula: an abnormal passage or opening between two structures in the body; may reflect breakdown of the incision line following palatal surgery.

Fricatives: consonant sounds produced when air is channeled through a small constriction in the mouth and becomes turbulent; includes *th, f, v, s, z, sh, zh,* and *h.*

Function words: words that are less crucial to the meaning of a sentence, such as articles (the, a).

Gene: the basic unit of heredity, which is made up of DNA and carries genetic information in each cell.

Genetic: referring to genes.

Gesture: a movement made as a nonverbal way of communicating.

Grammatical morphemes: parts of the sentence that are typically attached to nouns and verbs; they hold the main parts of the sentence together.

Hypernasality: excessive nasal resonance that may be heard during production of vowels and voiced consonants.

Hyponasality: insufficient nasal resonance during production of nasal consonants (*m, n, ng*), which can make a speaker sound as though he has a "stuffy" nose.

Incisors (central and lateral): the eight teeth in the front of the mouth (four on top and four on bottom).

Infant-directed speech: speech that is directed to babies that is different from the speech that we use when we talk to adults; it is higher pitched, contains shorter sentences, and is more directed to the "here and now."

Intentional communication: to communicate with a goal in mind.

Invented spelling: an early stage in learning to write when young children spell words in creative ways based on their early knowledge of sounds.

Jargon: a string of speech sounds produced by a baby that has the same intonation as a meaningful utterance but has no intelligible words.

Joint attention: to focus attention on an object or event with another person.

Mandible: the lower jaw bone.

Maxilla: the upper jaw bone.

Mirror-Map: a language learning technique in which an adult imitates a child's actions and uses words to describe the actions.

Modeling: a language learning technique in which an adult offers a sample for the child to imitate.

Myringotomy: a surgical procedure involving an incision in the eardrum.

Myringotomy tubes: plastic, metal, or Teflon tubes that are placed in the eardrum to keep the middle ear space aerated and prevent the accumulation of fluid. They are also called pressure equalization tubes (PE), ventilation tubes, or grommets.

Nasal emission: air flowing through the nose during production of pressure consonants when VPI is present; may be audible or inaudible.

Nasoalveolar molding: a nonsurgical treatment that reshapes the lip, gums, and nostrils prior to cleft lip and palate surgery to reduce the severity of the cleft.

Otitis media: inflammation of the middle ear; includes the following types:
- **Acute otitis media:** when the fluid in the middle ear becomes infected.
- **Otitis media with effusion:** a build-up of sticky fluid in the middle ear that is not infected.
- **Otitis externa:** occurs when water gets trapped in the outer ear and causes bacteria to grow.

Otolaryngologist: a physician who is trained in the diagnosis and treatment of diseases of the ear, nose, and throat; an ear, nose, and throat (ENT) specialist.

Otologic: related to the study, diagnosis, and treatment of diseases of the ear.

Palate: the roof of the mouth; made up of the hard and soft palate.

Palatoplasty: surgery on the palate.

Pharyngeal: referring to or coming from the throat.

Pharyngeal augmentation: a procedure for treating VPI that involves injecting or implanting a material into the back wall of the throat. The bulge in the back wall of the throat that is created by this material minimizes the distance that the palate must move to achieve velopharyngeal closure.

Pharyngeal flap: a flap of tissue raised from the back wall of the throat and attached to the soft palate.

Pharyngoplasty: surgery in the throat.

Pharynx: the throat.

Phonology: the study of speech sounds and the rules that govern them.

Phonological awareness: awareness of the individual sounds that make up words.

Premaxilla: the triangular piece of bone that houses the upper central and lateral incisors.

Pressure consonants: consonants that require high oral pressure for production; in English, they are the *stops* (*p, b, t, d, k, g*), *fricatives* (*f, v, s, z, sh, zh, th*), and *affricates* (*ch* and *j*).

Primary surgery: initial surgery to repair a cleft lip or cleft palate.

Print concepts: knowledge about books and how they are used for reading.

Prenatal: before birth.

Raspberries: vocalizations that babies make that sound like blowing air through closed lips.

Reflexive vocalizations: vocalizations related to the baby's physical state (e.g., coughing).

Resonance: referring to the increase in intensity of sound waves in a cavity; in speech, usually refers to the cavity (mouth or nose) where the most air is resonating.

Rhinoplasty: reconstruction of the nose.

Secondary surgery: surgery performed after original lip and/or palate surgeries to improve appearance or speech.

Sequence: one problem that causes other problems to occur.

Sibilants: fricative and affricate consonants produced by directing air toward the sharp edge of the teeth; they include *s, z, ch,* and *j.*

Soft palate: velum; makes up the back one-third of the roof of the mouth.

Sonogram: an image produced by ultrasound.

Speech perception: how the sounds of the language are heard and understood.

Speech recasting: a technique to promote speech sound development in which the adult repeats the child's words and emphasizes a sound in the word that was mispronounced by the child.

Sphincter pharyngoplasty: surgical procedure for VPI that involves taking flaps of tissue behind the tonsils and using them to line the back wall of the throat, thus bringing the back of the throat closer to the soft palate.

Stop (plosives) consonants: consonants produced by obstructing airflow in the mouth and then releasing it explosively; includes *p, b, t, d, k,* and *g.*

Submucous cleft: a cleft in the muscle in the soft palate; it is hidden from view by the mucous membrane (lining) of the roof of the mouth.

Syndrome: a combination of symptoms or problems that occur together and are associated with a particular disease or disorder.

Telegraphic speech: "sentences" that contain only the main ideas (nouns, verbs); the "little words" (articles) and grammatical forms are missing.

Tonsils: small masses of lymphatic tissue located on either side of the back of the mouth; part of the lymphatic system which assists in fighting infection. Tonsils may be removed if repeated infections occur or if their size hinders breathing.

Tympanometry: a test of middle ear function in which air pressure is applied to the eardrum to examine its mobility.

Turn-Taking: an early communication skill in which parent and child take turns communicating.

Unilateral: one sided.

Uvula: the small flap of tissue that hangs down from the back of the soft palate. The purpose of the uvula is not yet clear.

Velopharyngeal closure: separation of mouth and nose that occurs when the soft palate moves against the back wall of the throat.

Velopharyngeal inadequacy (VPI): inability to achieve velopharyngeal closure. Results in inappropriate nasal air flow and nasal-sounding speech.

Velum: the soft palate.

Vermilion: the red, fleshy portion of the lip.

Vocal play: when babies produce a variety of vowel- and consonant-like sounds including growls, squeals, and other noises that sound like they are "playing" with different sound patterns.

VPI: See velopharyngeal inadequacy.

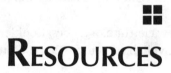

RESOURCES

The books, articles, and websites listed below offer information on speech-language development, cleft lip/palate, and related conditions. Unless otherwise noted in this book, we do not endorse any particular product or site.

▪▪ Articles, Booklets, and Fact Sheets

"About Antibiotic Use and Resistance." United States Centers for Disease Control and Prevention. http://www.cdc.gov/getsmart/ antibiotic-use/uri/ear-infection.html.

"Antibiotics for Middle-Ear Infection (Acute Otitis Media) in Children." The Cochrane Collaboration. http://www.cochrane.org. Venekamp, R. P., Sanders, S. I., Glasziou, P. P., Del Mar, C. B., & Rovers, M. M. (2013).

"As You Get Older." Cleft Palate Foundation. http://cleftline.org/ docs/Booklets/TEN-01.pdf. Print copies are also available from the Cleft Palate Foundation (see address below).

"Cleft Lip/Palate & Craniofacial Specialists in Your Area." www. cleftline.org/parents-individuals/team-care. Print copies are also available from the Cleft Palate Foundation (see address below).

"Cleft Surgery." www.cleftline.org/docs/Booklets/SUR-01.pdf. Print copies are also available from the Cleft Palate Foundation (see address below).

"Clinical Practice Guidelines: Otitis Media with Effusion." American Academy of Otolaryngology-Head and Neck Surgery. http:// www.entnet.org. Rosenfeld R. M., et al. (2004).

"Ear Infections in Children." National Institutes of Health–Institute on Deafness and Other Communication Disorders. http://www. nidcd.nih.gov/health/hearing/Pages/earinfections.aspx.

"Emergent Literacy: Early Reading and Writing Development." American Speech-Language-Hearing Association. http://www.asha. org/public/speech/emergent-literacy.htm. Roth, F. P., Paul, D. R., & Pierotti, A. M. (2006).

"Facts about Birth Defects." Centers for Disease Control and Prevention. www.cdc.gov/ncbddd/birthdefects/facts.html.

"Facts about Cleft Lip and Palate." Centers for Disease Control and Prevention. www.cdc.gov/ncbddd/birthdefects/CleftLip.html.

"Feeding Your Baby." (2009). Cleft Palate Foundation. http:// www.cleftline.org/parents/feeding_your_baby. Print copies are also available from the Cleft Palate Foundation (see address below).

"Feeding Infants: A Guide for Use in the Child Nutrition Programs." (2001). United States Department of Agriculture. http://www. fns.usda.gov/sites/default/files/feeding_infants.pdf.

"Genetics and You." (2001). Cleft Palate Foundation. www.cleftline. org/docs/Booklets/GEN-01.pdf. Print copies are also available from the Cleft Palate Foundation (see address below).

"Hearing Loss in Children." Centers for Disease Control and Prevention. http://www.cdc.gov/ncbddd/hearingloss/index.html.

"Let's Read about It." Cleft Palate Foundation. http://www.cleftline. org/parents-individuals/books/.

"Parameters for Evaluation and Treatment of Patients with Cleft Lip/ Palate or Other Craniofacial Anomalies. (2009). American Cleft Palate-Craniofacial Association. http://www.acpa-cpf.org/uploads/site/Parameters_Rev_2009.pdf. Print copies are also available from the American Cleft Palate-Craniofacial Association, 1504 East Franklin Street, Suite 102, Chapel Hill, NC 27514-2820.

"Prenatal Diagnosis of Cleft Lip and Cleft Palate." (2014). Cleft Palate Foundation. www.cleftline.org/wp-content/uploads/2012/03/ PRE-01.pdf. Print copies are also available from the Cleft Palate Foundation (see address below).

"Preparing Your Child for Social Situations." Cleft Palate Foundation. www.cleftline.org/docs/PDF_Factsheets/Social_Interaction.pdf. Print copies are also available from the Cleft Palate Foundation (see address below).

"Understanding Bullying." Centers for Disease Control. http://www. cdc.gov/violenceprevention/pdf/bullyingfactsheet2012-a.pdf.

▪▪ Books for Parents

Apel, K., and Masterson, J. (2001). *Beyond Baby Talk: From Sounds to Sentences: A Parent's Complete Guide to Language Development*. New York: Three Rivers Press.

Bardige, B. S. (2009). *Talk to Me, Baby!* Baltimore: Paul H. Brookes.

Dougherty, D. P. (2005). *Teach Me How to Say It Right*. Oakland, CA: New Harbinger Publications.

Gruman-Trinkler, C. T. (2001). *Your Cleft-Affected Child: The Complete Book of Information, Resources, and Hope*. Nashville: Turner Publishing.

Losee, J., Kirschner, R. E., Smith, D., Straub, A., and Lawrence, C. (2015). *Comprehensive Cleft Care: Family Edition*. Boca Raton, FL: CRC Press.

Lovegrove, E. (2006). *Help! I'm Being Bullied*. Pembrokeshire, UK: Accent Press Ltd.

▪▪ Books for Children and Teens

Below is a list of selected books that were written for or by children and adults with cleft lip and palate. We have also included a title (*Stand Tall, Molly Lou Melon*) that focuses on self-esteem and is a particular favorite of one of the authors.

Children

Chamberlain, K. (2009). *Early Articulation Books for Cleft Palate Speech* series. East Moline, IL: Linguasystems.

Graham, J. (2006). *A Special Smile*. Bloomington, IN: Trafford Publishing.

Johnson-Burnham, M. (2013). *Cleft Talk for Kids*. North Charleston, SC: CreateSpace Independent Publishing Platform.

Lovell, P., and Catrow, D. (2001). *Stand Tall, Molly Lou Melon*. New York: G.P. Putnam's Sons.

Peckinpah, S. (1993). *Rosey, The Imperfect Angel*. Westlake Village, CA: Dasan Productions.

Teens/Parents

Brown, I. B. (2011). *Before the Lark*. Lubbock, TX: Texas Tech University Press.

Burglehaus, M. T. (2002). *Stop Singing, People Might Hear You: My Cleft Book*. Calgary, Alberta: Maria T. Burglehaus Publishing.

Cwir, J.M. (2013). *I Wish I'd Known How Much I'd Love You*. www.iwishidknown.yolasite.com.

Palacio, R. J. (2012) *Wonder.* New York: Knopf.

Wilde, A.J. (2013). *White Bees.* www.amyjowilde.com

▪▪ Websites

American Speech-Language-Hearing Association (ASHA)
2200 Research Boulevard
Rockville, MD 20850-3289 USA
301-296-5700; 800-638-8255
http://www.asha.org/public/
　　This is a professional, credentialing association for audiologists and speech-language pathologists. They provide information to the public on hearing and balance, as well as speech-language development and disorders.

Ameriface
P.O. Box 751112
Las Vegas, NV 89136-1112
888-486-1209
info@ameriface.org
http://www.ameriface.org
　　This organization provides information and emotional support to individuals with facial differences and their families. They publish a monthly newsletter, the Cleft Advocate: www.cleftadvocate.org.

Center for Early Literacy Learning
info@puckett.org
http://www.earlyliteracylearning.org
　　This is a site funded by the US Department of Education that was developed for parents, teachers, researchers, and others interested in developing early language and literacy skills in children from birth to five years of age who are at risk for delays in development. Resources specifically for parents (http://www.earlyliteracylearning.org/parentresource1.php) include videos, downloadable podcasts, posters, and other materials that model a variety of activities, and are designed to promote literacy skills in infants, toddlers, and preschoolers. An outstanding resource for parents.

Cleft Palate Foundation
1504 East Franklin St., Suite 102
Chapel Hill, NC 27514-2820
616-329-1335; 800-242-5338
info@cleftline.org
http://www.cleftline.org www.cleftsmile.org
 The Cleft Palate Foundation (CPF) is an organization devoted to individuals with cleft lip/palate and other craniofacial conditions as well as their families. They provide a number of fact sheets and booklets on cleft lip/palate and other craniofacial conditions that can be downloaded from their website or ordered in print form. Many publications can be downloaded in Spanish as well as English. The CPF provides a booklet and videos with excellent feeding information. The organization also provides college scholarships for individuals with craniofacial differences.

FACES: The National Craniofacial Association
P.O. Box 11082
Chattanooga, TN 37401
423-266-1632; 800-332-2373
http://www.faces-cranio.org/
 This organization provides information and support for individuals with craniofacial conditions, and fosters public awareness of these conditions. It can also provide assistance with expenses associated with travel to a craniofacial center for assessment and surgery for individuals who meet specific financial and medical criteria.

The International 22Q Foundation
P.O. Box 2269
Voorhees, NJ 08077
877-739-1849
info@22q.org
http://www.22q.org
 This organization provides information and support for individuals with 22q, and fosters public awareness of these conditions.

Language Development in Internationally Adopted Children.
Sharon Glennen, Ph.D.
Towson University
Towson, MD 21252
 sglennen@towson.edu
http://pages.towson.edu/sglennen/index.htm.

This website provides information about language development for internationally adopted children. Pre-adoption questions are provided.

Stop Bullying
www.stopbullying.gov

This website defines the types of bullying that can occur and identifies strategies to prevent and respond to the problem.

Zero to Three
National Center for Infants, Toddlers, and Families
www.zerotothree.org

This website provides information about every aspect of your child's behavior and development (communication, social emotional, health, nutrition, sleep, play, etc.) from birth to age three years. In addition to print materials, the center offers podcasts and other interactive resources for parents and professionals.

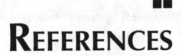

REFERENCES

American Academy of Otolaryngology-Head and Neck Surgery. http://www.entnet.org/.

American Academy of Pediatrics. http://www.aap.org/.

American Academy of Pediatrics. (2010). *Your baby's first year.* (3rd ed.). New York: Bantam Books.

American Cleft Palate-Craniofacial Association. (2009). *Parameters for evaluation and treatment of patients with cleft lip/palate or other craniofacial anomalies.* Chapel Hill, NC: American Cleft Palate-Craniofacial Association. http://www.acpa-cpf.org/up loads/site/Parameters_Rev_2009.pdf .

American Speech-Language-Hearing Association. (n.d.). Causes of hearing loss in children. Retrieved December 17, 2014 from http://www.asha.org/public/hearing/Causes-of-Hearing-Loss-in-Children.

Apel K., & Masterson, J. (2001). *Beyond baby talk: From sounds to sentences: A parent's complete guide to language development.* New York: Three Rivers Press.

Arosarena, O. A. (2007). Cleft lip and palate. *Otolaryngologic Clinics of North America, 40,* 27–60.

Arvedson J.C., & Brodsky, L. (2002). *Pediatric swallowing and feeding.* Albany, NY: Singular Publishing Group.

Austin, A. A., Druschel, C. M., Tyler, M. C., Romitti, P. A., West, I. I., Damiano, P. C., Robbins, J. M., & Burnett, W. (2010). Interdisciplinary craniofacial teams compared with individual providers: Is orofacial cleft care more comprehensive and do parents perceive better outcomes? *Cleft Palate-Craniofacial Journal, 47,* 1–8.

Bardige, B. S. (2009). *Talk to me, baby!* Baltimore: Paul H. Brookes.

Bernheim, N., Georges, M., Malevez, C., De Mey, A., & Mansbach, A. (2006). Embryology and epidemiology of cleft lip and palate. *B-ENT,* 11–19.

Browning, G. G., Rovers, M. M., Williamson, I., Lous, J., & Burton, M. J. (2010). Grommets (ventilation tubes) for hearing loss associated with otitis media with effusion in children. *Cochrane Database of Systematic Reviews, 2010.* Art. No.: CD001801. DOI: 10.1002/14651858.CD001801.pub3.

Catts, H., Fey, M., Tomblin, B., & Zhang, X. (2002). A longitudinal investigation of reading outcomes in children with language impairments. *Journal of Speech, Language, and Hearing Research, 45,* 1142–1157.

Centers for Disease Control and Prevention. (2014). Facts about cleft lip and palate. Retrieved December 9, 2014 from http://www.cdc.gov/ncbddd/birthdefects/CleftLip.html.

Centers for Disease Control and Prevention. (2015). Get smart: Know when antibiotics work. http://www.cdc.gov/getsmart/antibiotic-use/uri/ear-infection.html.

Chapman, K., Hardin-Jones, M., Goldstein, J., Halter, K. A., Havlik, R., & Schulte, J. (2008). Timing of palatal surgery and speech outcomes. *Cleft Palate-Craniofacial Journal, 45*(3), 297–308.

Chapman, K. L. (2011). The relationship between early reading skills and speech and language performance in young children with cleft lip and palate. *Cleft Palate-Craniofacial Journal, 48,* 301–211.

Cleft Palate Foundation. (2014). Feeding your baby. Retrieved from http:// www.cleftline.org/ parents/ feeding_your_baby.

Cleft Palate Foundation. (2001). Genetics and you (2nd ed.). Retrieved from www.cleftline.org/docs/Booklets/GEN-01.pdf.

Conboy, B. T. (2012). Language procession and production in infants and toddlers. In B. Goldstein (Ed.), *Bilingual language development & disorders in Spanish-English Speakers* (pp. 47–71). Baltimore: Paul H. Brookes.

Cutler-Landsman, D. (2007). *Educating children with velo-cardio-facial syndrome.* San Diego: Plural Publishing.

Dailey, S. (2013). Feeding and swallowing management in infants with cleft and craniofacial anomalies. *Perspectives on Speech Science and Orofacial Disorders, 23,* 62–72.

Dixon, M. J., Marazita, M. L., Beaty, T. H., and Murray, J. C. (2011). Cleft lip and palate: Understanding genetic and environmental influences. *Nature Reviews Genetics, 12,* 167–178.

Gildersleeve-Newman, C. E., Kester, E. S., Davis, B. L., & Pena, E. P. (2008). English speech sound development in preschool-aged children from bilingual English-Spanish environments. *Speech, Language, and Hearing Services in the Schools, 39,* 314–328.

Gindis, B. (2003). What should adoptive parents know about their child's language-based school difficulties? BG Center Online School, Post-Adoption Learning Center. http://www.adoption-articlesdirectory.com/.

Glennen, S. (2008, December 16). Speech and language "myth-busters" for internationally adopted children. *The ASHA Leader*.

Glennen, S. (2007). Predicting language outcomes for internationally adopted children, *Journal of Speech, Language and Hearing Research, 50*, 529–548.

Glennen, S. (2014). A longitudinal study of language and speech in children who were internationally adopted at different ages, *Language, Speech, and Hearing in the Schools, 45,* 185-293.

Groher, M. E., & Crary, M. A. (2010). Dysphagia: Clinical management in adults and children. Maryland Heights, MO: Mosby.

Hansson, E., Svensson, H., & Becker, M. (2012). Adopted children with cleft lip or palate, or both, require special needs cleft surgery. *Journal Plastic Hand Surgery, 46*, 75–79.

Hardin-Jones, M. A., & Jones, D. L. (2005). Speech production of preschoolers with cleft palate. *Cleft Palate-Craniofacial Journal, 42*, 7–13.

Hardin-Jones, M. A., Chapman, K. L., Wright, J., Halter, K.A., Schulte, J., Dean, J. Havlik, R. J., & Goldstein, J. (2002). The impact of early palatal obturation on consonant development in babies with unrepaired cleft palate. *Cleft Palate-Craniofacial Journal, 39*, 157–163.

Hirsh-Pasek, K., & Golinkoff, R. (2003). Einstein never used flash cards. New York, NY: St. Martin's Press.

Hoff, E. (2009). *Language development* (4th ed). Belmont, CA: Wadsworth/Cengage Learning.

Iglesias, A., & Rojas, R. (2012). Bilingual language development of English language learners: Modeling the growth of two languages. In B. Goldstein (Ed.), *Bilingual language development & disorders in Spanish-English speakers* (pp. 3–30). Baltimore: Paul H. Brookes.

Isaacson, J. E., & Vora, N. M. (2003). Differential diagnosis and treatment of hearing loss. *American Family Physician, 68*(6), 1125–1132.

Johnston, J. C., Durieux-Smith, A., & Bloom, K. (2005). Teaching gestural signs to infants to advance child development: A review of the evidence. *First Language, 25*(2), 235–251.

Justice, L. M. (2006). *Clinical approaches to emergent literacy intervention.* San Diego, CA: Plural.

Kaderavek, J., & Justice, L. (2004). Embedded-explicit emergent literacy intervention II: Goal selection and implementation in early childhood classrooms. *Language, Speech, and Hearing Services in Schools, 36,* 251–263.

Katzel, B. A., Basile, P., Koltz, P. F., Marcus, J. R., & Girotto, J. A. (2009). Current surgical practices in cleft care: Cleft palate repair techniques and postoperative care. *Plastic and Reconstructive Surgery, 124,* 899–906.

Kohli, S. S., & and Kohli, V. S. (2012). A comprehensive review of the genetic basis of cleft lip and palate. *Journal of Oral and Maxillofacial Pathology, 16*(X), 64–72.

Kohnert, K., & Derr, A. (2012). Language intervention with bilingual children. In B. Goldstein (Ed.), *Bilingual language development & disorders in Spanish-English speakers* (pp. 337–356). Baltimore: Paul H. Brookes.

Language minority school age children. (2009). Washington, DC: National Center for Education Statistics.

Lieberthal, A. S., et al. (2013, March 1). Clinical practice guideline: The diagnosis and treatment of acute otitis media. *Pediatrics, 131*(3), e964–e999.

Lonigan, C. J., & Whitehurst, G. J. (1998). Relative efficacy of parent and teacher involvement in shared-reading intervention for preschool children from low-income backgrounds. *Early Childhood Research Quarterly, 13*(2), 263–290.

McDonald, S., Langton Hewer, C. D., & Nunez, D. A. (2008). Grommets (ventilation tubes) for recurrent acute otitis media in children. *Cochrane Database of Systematic Reviews 2008,* Issue 4. Art. No.: CD004741. DOI: 10.1002/14651858.CD004741.pub2.

McGuinness, D. (2003). Growing a reader from birth. New York, NY: W. W. Norton & Company.

McLean, J., & Synder-McLean. L. (1999). How children learn language. San Diego: Singular Publishing.

McWilliams, L. (2006). Integrating phonological sensitivity and oral language instruction into enhanced dialogic reading. In L. A. Justice. (Ed.), *Clinical approaches to emergent literacy intervention.* (pp. 261–294). San Diego, CA: Plural Publishing.

Merritt, L. (2005). Part 1: Understanding the embryology and genetics of cleft lip and palate. *Advances in Neonatal Care,* 5, 64–71.

Miller, I. (2000). Initial assessment of growth, development, and the effects of institutionalization in internationally adopted children. *Pediatric Annuals, 29,* 224–232.

Moller, K.T., Starr, C. D., and Johnson, S. A. (1990). *A parent's guide to cleft lip and palate.* Minneapolis: University of Minnesota Press.

Molofsky, A. J., & Blum-Kemelor, D. M. (2001). *Feeding infants: A guide for use in the child nutrition programs.* Washington, DC: US Department of Agriculture. http://www.fns.usda.gov/sites/default/files/feeding_infants.pdf.

Nathani, S., & Stark, R. (1996). Can conditioning procedures yield representative infant vocalizations in the laboratory? *First Language, 16,* 365–387.

O'Gara, M. M., and Logeman, J. A. (1988). Phonetic analysis of the speech development of babies with cleft palate. *Cleft Palate Journal, 25,* 122–134.

Owens, R. (2012). *Language development: An introduction* (8th ed.). Saddle River, NJ: Pearson.

Palacios, J., Roman, M., & Camacho, C. (2010). Growth and development in internationally adopted children: Extent and timing of recovery after early adversity. *Child: Care, Health and Development, 37* (2), 282–288.

Paul, R., & Norbury, C. (2012). *Language disorders from infancy through adolescence: Listening, speaking, reading, writing, and communicating.* (4th ed.). St. Louis: Elsevier.

Peterson-Falzone, S. J., Hardin-Jones, M. A., & Karnell, M. P. (2010). *Cleft palate speech* (4th ed.). St. Louis: Mosby.

Ponduri, S., Bradley, R., Ellis, P. E., Brookes, S. T., Sandy, J. R., & Ness, A. R. (2009). The management of otitis media with early routine insertion of grommets in children with cleft palate: A systematic review. *Cleft Palate-Craniofacial Journal, 46,* 30–38.

Prahl, C., Kuijpers-Jagtman, M. A., Vant Hof, M.A., & Prahl-Andersen, B. (2005). Infant orthopedics in UCLP: Effect on feeding, weight, and length: A randomized clinical trial (Dutchcleft). *Cleft Palate-Craniofacial Journal, 42,* 171–177.

Preparing your child for social situations. Cleft Palate Foundation. Retrieved December 16, 2014 from www.cleftline.org/docs/ PDF_Factsheets/Social_Interaction.pdf.

Redford-Badwal, D. A., Mabry, K., Frassinelli, J. D. (2003). Impact of cleft lip and palate on nutritional health and oral-motor development. *The Dental Clinics of North America, 47,* 305–317.

Reid, J., Kilpatrick, N., & Reilly, S. (2006). A prospective, longitudinal study of feeding skills in a cohort of babies with cleft conditions. *Cleft Palate-Craniofacial Journal, 43,* 702–709.

Robbins, J. M., Damiano, P., Druschei, C. M., Hobbs, C.A., Romitti, P. A., Austin, A .A., Tyler, M., Reading, A., & Burnett, W. (2010). Prenatal diagnosis of orofacial clefts: Association with maternal satisfaction, team care, and treatment outcomes. *Cleft Palate-Craniofacial Journal, 47,* 476–481.

Roberts, J. E., & Ziesel, S. A. (2000). Ear infections and language development. Published in collaboration with ASHA and the National Center for Early Development & Learning. Available at http://fpg.unc.edu/resources/ear-infections-and-language-development.

Roberts, J. E., Rosenfeld, R. M., & Zeisel, S. A. (2004). Otitis media and speech and language: A meta-analysis of prospective studies. *Pediatrics, 113*(3), 238–248.

Roberts, J. A., Pollack, K. E., Krakow, R., Price, J., Fulmer, K. C., & Wang, P. P. (2005). Language development in preschool-age children adopted from China. *Journal of Speech, Language, Hearing Research, 48,* 93–107.

Rosenfeld, R. M., Schwartz, S. R., Cannon, C. R., Roland, P. S., Simon, G. R., Kumar, K. A., & Robertson, P. J. (2014). Clinical practice guideline: Acute otitis externa executive summary. *Otolaryngology—Head and Neck Surgery,* 150(2), 161–168.

Rosin, P. (2006). Literacy intervention in a culturally and linguistically diverse world: The linking language and literacy project. In L. M. Justice (Ed.), *Clinical approaches to emergent literacy intervention* (pp. 391–438). San Diego, CA: Plural Publishing.

Rvachew, S., & Brosseau-Lapre, F. (2012). *Developmental phonological disorders: Foundations of clinical practice.* San Diego, CA: Plural Publishing.

Sadove, A. S., Eppley, B. L., Jones, D. L., & Hardin-Jones, M. (1998). Velopharyngeal insufficiency. In M. L. Bentz, *Pediatric plastic surgery*. Stamford, CT: Appleton and Lange.

Scherer, N. J., & Kaiser, A. (2010). Enhanced milieu teaching/phonological emphasis: Application for children with cleft lip and palate. In L. Williams & R. McCauley (Eds.), *Speech sound disorders in children*. Baltimore: Paul H. Brookes.

Scherer, N. J., Boyce, S., & Martin, G. (2013). Pre-linguistic children with cleft palate: Growth of gesture, vocalization, and word use. *International Journal of Speech-Language Pathology, 15,* 586–592.

Scherer, N. J., Kaiser, A., & Totino, L. (2012). Speech-language skills in young internationally adopted children with repaired cleft palate. Poster at the American Speech-Language-Hearing Association Convention, Atlanta.

Schwartz, R. G., Chapman, K., Prelock, P. A., Terrell, B. Y., & Rowan, L. E. (1985). Facilitation of early syntax through discourse structure. *Journal of Child Language, 12,* 13–26.

Schwartz, R. G., Chapman, K., Terrell, B., & Rowan, L. (1985). Facilitating word combination in language-impaired children through discourse structure. *Journal of Speech and Hearing Disorders, 50,* 31–40.

Schwartz, S., & Heller, J. E. (1996). *The new language of toys: Teaching communication skills to children with special need*. Bethesda, MD: Woodbine House.

Shkoukani, M.A., Chen, M., & Vong, A. (2013). Cleft lip: A comprehensive review. *Frontiers in Pediatrics, 1,* 53.

Shprintzen, R. J., & Golding-Kushner, K. (2008). *Velo-cardio-facial syndrome: Volume I.* San Diego: Plural Publishing.

Snedeker, J., Geren, J., & Shafto, C. L. (2007). Starting over: International adoption as a natural experiment in language development. *Psychological Science, 18*(1), 79–87.

Snyder, L., & Scherer, N. (2004). The development of symbolic play and language in toddlers with cleft palate. *American Journal of Speech Language Pathology,13,* 66–80.

Sullivan, S., Jung, Y., & Mulliken, J. B. (2014). Outcomes of cleft palatal repair for internationally adopted children. *Plastic and Reconstructive Surgery,* 1445–1452.

Swanson, J., Smartt, J., Saltzman, B., Birgfeld, C., Hopper, R., Gruss, J., & Tse, R. (2014). Adopted children with cleft lip and/or palate: A unique and growing population. *Plastic & Reconstructive Surgery, 143*(2), 183e–193e.

Tan, T. X., & Yang, Y. (2005). Language development of Chinese adoptees 18–35 months old. *Early Childhood Research Quarterly, 20,* 57–68.

Tan, S.P., Greene, A. K., & Mulliken, J. B. (2012). Current surgical management of bilateral cleft lip in North America. *Plastic Reconstructive Surgery, 129*(6), 1347–1355.

Venekamp, R. P., Sanders, S., Glasziou, P. P., Del Mar, C. B., & Rovers, M. M. (2013). Antibiotics for acute otitis media in children. *Cochrane Database of Systematic Reviews 2013,* Issue 1. Art. No.: CD000219. DOI: 10.1002/14651858.CD000219.pub3.

VPI Surgical Trial Group (2005). Pharyngeal flap and sphincterplasty for velopharyngeal insufficiency have equal outcomes at 1 year postoperatively: Results of a randomized trial. *Cleft Palate-Craniofacial Journal, 42,* 501–511.

Wilson, S. (2009). Attending to relationships: Attachment formation within families of internationally adopted children. *Topics in Language Disorders, 29*(2), 18–31.

Young, S. E. L., Purcell, A. A., Ballard, K. J., Liow, S. J. R., Silva Ramos, S. D., S., & Heard, R. (2012). Bilingual children with nonsyndromic cleft lip and/or palate: Language and memory skills. *Journal of Speech, Language, and Hearing Research, 55,* 1314–1328.

INDEX

■ About the Authors

Mary Hardin-Jones is a Professor in the Division of Communication Disorders at the University of Wyoming. She has served on cleft palate teams in several different states throughout her career and has been actively involved in research studying speech production of children with cleft lip and palate for over thirty years. Dr. Hardin-Jones is particularly interested in early speech development and treatment outcomes for these children. She has co-authored two textbooks and has numerous presentations and publications pertaining to these topics. Dr. Hardin-Jones is a Fellow of the American Speech-Language-Hearing Association.

Kathy Chapman is a Professor in the Department of Communication Sciences and Disorders at the University of Utah. Her research has focused on describing the speech and language development of infants and preschoolers with cleft palate. She is currently involved in the first inter-center comparison of speech outcomes for children with cleft palate to be carried out in the United States. Her research has been funded by the National Institutes of Health. Dr. Chapman has numerous research articles, book chapters, and national and international presentations related to her work with young children with cleft palate. Dr. Chapman is a Fellow of the American Speech-Language-Hearing Association.

Nancy J. Scherer is Professor and Chair of the Speech and Hearing Science department at Arizona State University. Her research and clinical interests have addressed the assessment of speech and language development of children with cleft lip and palate and other craniofacial conditions, and models of early intervention for children with cleft lip and/or palate, including strategies for parents and healthcare professionals in early speech and language intervention. In addition to intervention models, her research has emphasized prevention of speech and language delays through early identification and parent training. Dr. Scherer is a Fellow of the American Speech-Language-Hearing Association.